THE GLYCEMIC INDEX DIET

A Guide to Managing Diabetes through a Low - GI Diet

Bonus: 30 Day Meal Planner

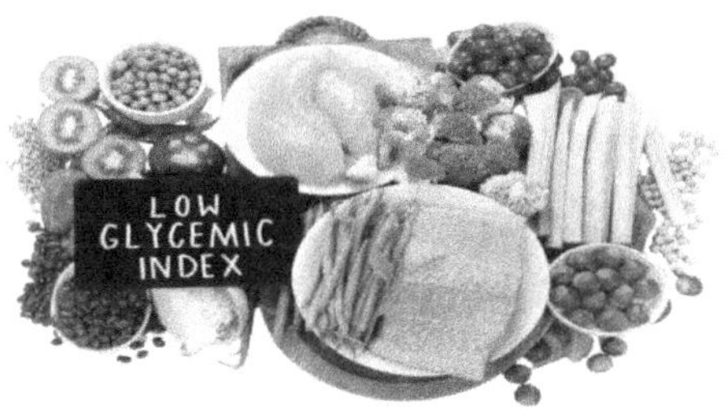

BENJAMIN AARON

Copyright © 2022 by Benjamin Aaron

GAIN ACCESS TO MORE BOOKS FROM ME

TABLE OF CONTENTS

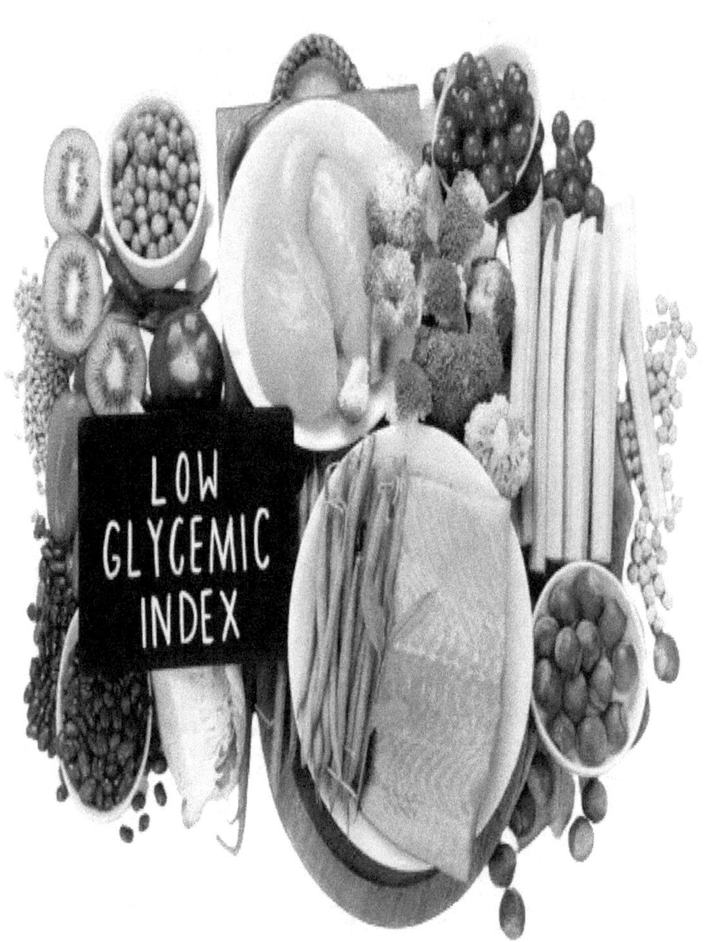
LOW
GLYCEMIC
INDEX

CHAPTER 1

INTRODUCTION

Olivia had been living with diabetes for the past five years, and she had tried many different treatments to try and reverse it. She had tried medications, insulin injections, and even the latest cutting-edge treatments, but nothing seemed to make a difference.

One day, while surfing the internet, Olivia came across an article and clicked on the link about a new approach to reversing diabetes: a low glycemic index diet. She made the decision to test it, and she was astonished by the outcomes. She started eating more whole grains, vegetables, and fruits, and she cut out processed foods and sugary snacks.

Within a few weeks, Olivia noticed her blood sugar levels were lower and more stable. After a few months, her doctor was astonished to find that her diabetes had disappeared completely.

Olivia was thrilled. She had finally been able to reverse her diabetes without any medications or injections. She was so happy that she had discovered the power of a low glycemic index diet, and she was eager to share her success story with others.

GLYCEMIC INDEX DIET

The Glycemic Index Diet is a powerful tool that can help you take control of your health and achieve your weight goals. By understanding the glycemic index, you can make the right food choices to keep your blood sugar levels in check and improve your overall health. This diet is based on the concept of the glycemic index, which is a measure of how quickly a food raises your blood sugar levels. The glycemic index ranks foods on a scale from 0 to 100, with higher numbers indicating a greater impact on your blood sugar levels. By selecting foods with lower glycemic indexes, you can improve your health, lose weight, and reduce your risk of chronic diseases such as diabetes, heart disease, and certain types of cancer. So, if you're ready to take control of your health and reach your weight goals, the Glycemic Index Diet may be the right choice for you.

The glycemic index diet is a diet that is based on how foods affect the body's blood sugar levels. This diet is often recommended for people with diabetes, as it helps to regulate blood sugar levels and can help to prevent some of the health complications associated with diabetes. The glycemic index diet focuses on choosing low-glycemic foods, which are foods that are slowly digested and absorbed, and therefore have a minimal impact on blood sugar levels. Foods that are high in fiber, protein, and healthy fats are encouraged on the glycemic index diet, as they help to slow digestion and the release of glucose into the bloodstream. Eating meals and snacks that contain a combination of these foods can help to keep blood sugar levels stable throughout the day.

By following a glycemic index diet, people with diabetes can better manage their blood sugar levels and reduce their risk of developing diabetes-related complications. In addition, this diet is beneficial for those looking to lose weight, as it emphasizes nutritious and low-glycemic foods that can help to reduce cravings and keep you feeling fuller for longer.

The glycemic index diet is an important tool for people with diabetes and those looking to improve their health. By choosing foods that are low on the glycemic index and eating them in combination with healthy fats and proteins, you can help to regulate your blood sugar levels and lower your chance of acquiring problems from diabetes.

With careful planning, the glycemic index diet can be a successful and effective way to maintain good health.

Let's get started!

WHAT IS DIABETES?

Diabetes Mellitus is a chronic, metabolic disease (disorder) characterized by elevated levels of blood glucose (or blood sugar). It prevents the body from utilizing glucose completely or partially and characterized by raised glucose concentratioin in the blood and alteration in carbohydrate, protein, and fat metabolism. It is caused by either inadequate insulin production or a lack of response to insulin in the body. Insulin is a hormone produced in the pancreas that helps to regulate the amount of sugar in the blood. When there is too much sugar in the blood, it can cause a number of health complications. Diabetes affects millions of people worldwide and can cause serious health complications, including heart disease, stroke, kidney disease, and nerve damage.

SYMPTOMS OF DIABETES

The most common symptoms of diabetes include increased thirst (Polydipsia) and urination (Polyruia), fatigue, difficulty losing weight, increased hunger (Polyphagia), and blurred vision (diabetic retinopathy).

People with diabetes may also experience skin problems (priuritis), such as itching, dryness, and slow-healing wounds. Nerve pain, tingling, and numbness in the hands and feet can also be a sign of diabetes.

Increased thirst and urination are one of the earliest signs of diabetes. People with diabetes may feel an increased thirst and a need to drink more fluids than usual. This is because the body is trying to rid itself of excess sugar by excreting it through the urine. People with diabetes may also notice they are urinating more often, as the body tries to clear the excess sugar from the bloodstream.

Fatigue is another common symptom of diabetes. This is because the body is not able to process and use the glucose in the blood as effectively as it should, leading to an overall feeling of tiredness and exhaustion.

Difficulty losing weight is another symptom of diabetes, as the body is not able to break down the sugar in the blood and use it for energy. This can lead to weight gain, even when following a healthy diet and exercise plan.

Increased hunger is another common symptom of diabetes. This is because the body is not able to properly utilize the sugar in the blood for energy, leaving the person feeling hungry more often than usual.

Blurred vision is one of the most serious symptoms of diabetes. This is because high levels of glucose in the blood can cause damage to the tiny blood vessels in the eyes, leading to vision problems.

Other possible symptoms occur as the uncontrolled condition become more serious. Diabetic nephropathy (Kidney problem), Fluid and electrolyte imbalance, Acidoisis (Ketosis, Ketonuria: due to increased fat metabolism), and eventually coma.

Diabetes is a serious condition that can lead to a number of health complications if left untreated. If you think you may have diabetes, it is important to see your doctor right away.

Eating right is also vital if you're trying to prevent or control diabetes. While exercise is also important, what you eat has the biggest impact when it comes to weight loss. But what does eating right for diabetes mean? Follow through this book as we unveil to you that no special foods or complicated diets are necessary.

DIAGNOSING DIABETES

Diabetes is a chronic condition that occurs when the body is unable to produce or use insulin properly, leading to high blood sugar levels. In order to diagnose diabetes, a healthcare provider must perform certain tests.

The first test is a fasting blood glucose test, which measures the amount of glucose in the blood after the patient has gone without food or drink for at least 8 hours. If the results are above the normal range, it may indicate diabetes.

The second test is an oral glucose tolerance test, which measures blood glucose levels after the patient has consumed a specific amount of glucose. If the results are above the normal range, it may also indicate diabetes.

The third test is a hemoglobin A1C test, which measures the average amount of glucose in the blood over the past 3 months. If the results are above the normal range, it may indicate diabetes.

Finally, a healthcare provider may also use urine tests or physical exams to diagnose diabetes.

If any of the tests mentioned above indicate diabetes, the healthcare provider may recommend additional tests such as an eye exam, a kidney function test, or a cholesterol test to help confirm the diagnosis.

Diabetes is a serious condition that requires proper management and treatment. Therefore, it is important to receive an accurate diagnosis in order to receive the necessary care.

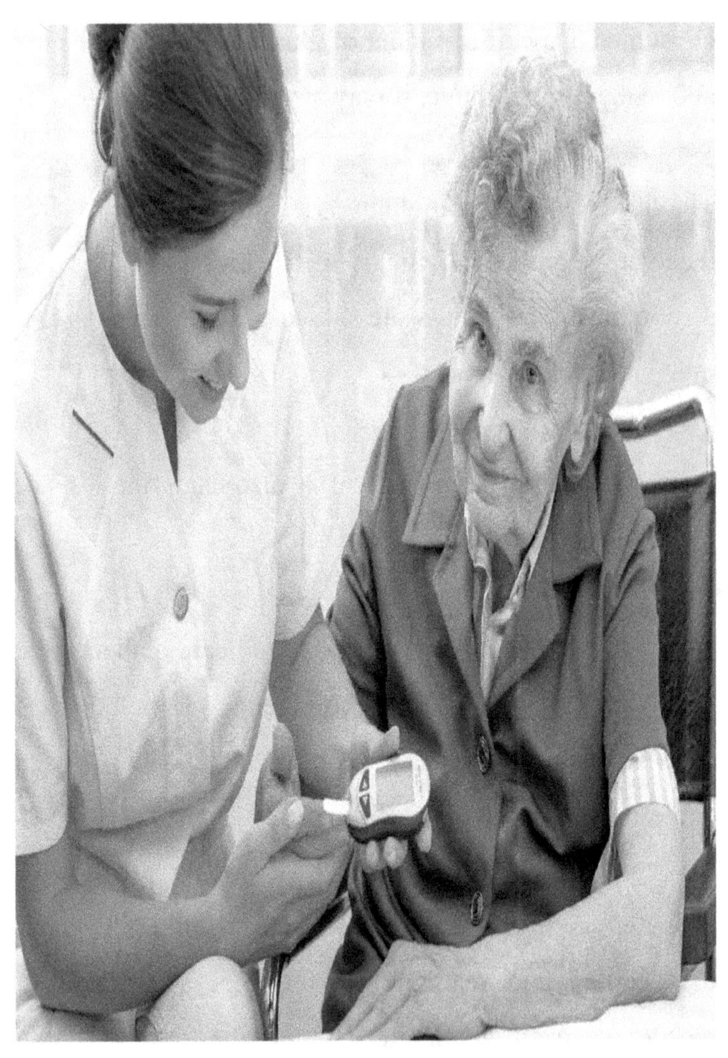

CHAPTER 2

HOW CAN THE GLYCEMIC INDEX DIET HELP?

The Glycemic Index Diet is a form of eating that focuses on selecting foods based on their glycemic index (GI) value. GI measures how quickly food is converted to glucose (sugar) in the body. Foods with a low GI value are slowly converted to glucose, while foods with a high GI value are quickly converted to glucose. This diet is based on the idea that eating low GI foods helps to maintain steady blood sugar levels, which in turn can help with weight loss, improved mood and energy levels, and better overall health. The main premise of the diet is to focus on eating low-GI foods, such as whole grains, fruits, vegetables, and dairy products, while avoiding high GI foods, such as white bread, processed foods, and sugary snacks. Additionally, the diet encourages reducing portion sizes, eating regular meals, and including some physical activity. This diet is not a strict meal plan, but instead offers guidelines for selecting healthy foods. Following the Glycemic Index Diet can help you maintain your health while still enjoying your favorite foods.

Overall, the Glycemic Index Diet is a beneficial way of eating that focuses on eating low GI foods to maintain steady blood sugar levels and support overall health.

By following the Glycemic Index Diet, you can enjoy the benefits of improved mood, energy levels, and weight loss while still enjoying your favorite foods.

BENEFITS OF GLYCEMIC INDEX DIET

1. **Improved Blood Sugar Control:** The glycemic index diet helps in controlling blood sugar levels by focusing on foods with a lower glycemic index. This can result in lower and more stable blood sugar levels.

2. **Reduced Risk of Complications:** Following a glycemic index diet may reduce the risk of developing complications associated with diabetes, including neuropathy, retinopathy, and heart disease.

3. **Increased Energy Levels:** Eating foods with a low glycemic index can help to keep blood sugar levels stable, which can lead to increased energy levels.

4. **Weight Loss:** Following a glycemic index diet can help to reduce body weight, which can help to improve overall health and reduce the risk of developing diabetes-related complications.

5. **Improved Cardiovascular Health:** Eating foods with a low glycemic index can reduce the risk of developing cardiovascular disease.

6. **Improved Mental Health:** Eating foods with a low glycemic index can also help to improve mental health, as they can reduce the risk of developing depression and anxiety.

7. **Reduced Risk of Diabetes:** Eating a diet low in glycemic index foods can reduce the risk of developing type 2 diabetes.

8. **Improved Digestion:** Eating foods with a low glycemic index can help to improve digestion and reduce the risk of developing gastrointestinal issues.

9. **Reduced Cravings:** Eating foods with a low glycemic index can help to reduce cravings, which can

help to reduce calorie intake and weight gain.

10. **Improved Nutrition:** Eating foods with a low glycemic index can help to ensure good nutrition, as they are typically high in fiber, vitamins, and minerals.

11. **Reduced Risk of Cancer:** Eating a diet low in glycemic index foods can reduce the risk of developing certain types of cancer.

12. **Reduced Risk of Age-Related Diseases:** Eating a diet low in glycemic index foods can reduce the risk of developing age-related diseases, such as Alzheimer's disease, Parkinson's disease, and dementia.

13. **Improved Quality of Life:** Improved blood sugar control, increased energy levels, and improved mental health can all lead to an improved quality of life.

14. **Reduced Risk of Osteoporosis:** Eating a diet low in glycemic index foods can reduce the risk of developing osteoporosis.

15. **Reduced Risk of Metabolic Syndrome:** Eating a diet low in glycemic index foods can reduce the risk of developing metabolic syndrome.

P.S: High intake of glycemic index foods could be detrimental to health because it pushes the body to extremes. This is especially true if one is overweight and sedentary, switching to eating mainly low glycemic index foods that slowly trickle glucose into blood streams keeps energy levels balanced and this means the subject will conserve energy extensively between meals. Additionally, low glycemic index food increases the body sensitivity to insulin. Low glycemic index diets, improve diabetes management. Besides, it reduces the risk of heart diseases and help people to lose and manage weight.

GLYCEMIC INDEX REFERENCE RANGE

Glycemic index food reference ranges from:

High Glycemic Index	70 – 100
Moderate Glycemic Index	55 – 70
Low Glycemic Index	< 55

GLYCEMIC INDEX OF COMMON FOODS

The table below shows the Glycemic Indices of some common foods.

Cereal Grains		
Rice Krispies	High	82
Cornflakes	High	83
Wheat Kernels	Low	41
Rice, Instant	Low	46
Rice, Parboiled	Low	48
Barley, Cracked	Low	50
Rice, browned	Medium	55
Rice, white	Medium	58
Barley, flakes	Medium	68
Millet	High	71
Diary Foods		
Yogurt low-fat (sweetened)	Low	14
Milk, Chocolate	Low	24
Milk - Fat free	Low	32
Milk – skimmed	Low	32
Milk semi – skimmed	Low	34

Ice cream (low fat)	Low	50
Ice cream	Medium	61

Fruits

Cherries	Low	22
Grape	Low	25
Apricots (dried)	Low	31
Apples	Low	38
Pears	Low	38
Oranges	Low	44
Grapes	Low	46
Bananas	Low	54
Mangoes	Medium	56
Pineapples	Medium	66
Watermelon	High	72
Potatoes, micro waved	High	82
Potatoes, instant	High	83
Potatoes, baked	High	85
Parnips	High	97

Snack Food and Sweet

Peanuts	Low	15
Snickers bar	Low	40

Chocolate bar, 30g	Low	49
Jams and marmalades	Low	49
Crisps	Low	54
Popcorn	Medium	55
Table Sugar (Sucrose)	Medium	65
Corn chips	High	74
Dates	High	103

Soups

Tomatoes soup, tinned	Low	38
Black bean soup, tinned	Medium	64

Pasta

Spaghetti, protein enriched	Low	27
Spaghetti whole wheat	Low	37
Spaghetti, white	Low	41
Macaroni	Low	45
Spaghetti, durum wheat	Medium	55
Macaroni cheese	Medium	64
Rice pasta, brown	High	92

Root Crop

Carrots, cooked	Low	39
Yam	Low	51

Sweet potatoes	Low	54
Potatoes, boiled	Medium	56
Potato, new	Medium	57
Potato, tinned	Medium	61
Beetroot	Medium	64
Potato steamed	Medium	65
Potato mashed	Medium	70
Chips	High	75
Green pea soup, tinned	Medium	66

Vegetable and Beans

Asparagus	Low	15
Cucumber	Low	15
Eggplant	Low	15
Green beans	Low	15
Lettuce, all varieties	Low	15
Spinach	Low	15
Tomatoes	Low	15
Soya beans	Low	18
Soya beans, boiled	Low	16
Peas, dried	Low	22
Kidney beans, boiled	Low	29

Lentils green, boiled	Low	29
Haricot beans, boiled	Low	38
Black – eyed beans	Low	41
Low-fat yogurt artificially sweetened	Low	15
Peppers, all varieties	Low	15
Baked beans, tinned	Low	48
Kidney beans, tinned	Low	52
Lentils green, tinned	Low	52
Bread beans	High	79

Biscuits

Showbread	Medium	64
Water biscuit	Medium	65
Rice cakes	High	77

Breads

Multi-grain bread	Low	48
Whole grain	Low	50
Pizza, cheese	Medium	60
Hamburger bun	Medium	61

MAKING THE GLYCEMIC INDEX EASY

What foods is slow-release? Several tools have been

designed to help answer this question. The glycemic index (GI) tells you how quickly a food turns into sugar in your system. Glycemic load looks at both the glycemic index and the amount of carbohydrate in a food, giving you a more accurate idea of how a food may affect your blood sugar level. High GI foods spike your blood sugar rapidly, while low GI foods have the least effect.

Foods can also be classified into three broad categories: fire, water, and coal. The harder your body needs to work to break down, the better.

Fire foods have a high GI, and are low in fiber and protein. They include 'White foods' (white rice, white pasta, white bread, potatoes, and most baked foods), sweets, chips, and many processed foods. They should be limited in your diet.

Water foods are free foods – meaning you can eat as many as you like. They include all vegetables and most types of fruits (fruit juice, dried fruit, and canned packed in syrup spike blood sugar quickly and are not considered water foods).

Coal foods have a low GI and are high in fibre and protein; they include nuts and seeds, lean meats, seafood, whole grains, and beans. They also include 'white food' replacements such as brown rice, whole-wheat bread, and whole-wheat.

PRINCIPLES OF LOW-GLYCEMIC EATING

1.   Eat a lot of non-starchy vegetables, beans, and fruits such as apples, pears, peaches, and berries. Even tropical fruits like bananas and papayastend to have a lower glycemic index than typical desserts.

2.   Eat grains in the least-processed state possible: "unbroken", such as whole –kernel bread, brown rice, and whole barley, millet, and wheat berries; or traditionally processed, such as stone-ground bread. Steel-cut oats and natural granola or muesli breakfast cereals.

3.   Limit whole potatoes and refined grain products such as white bread and white pasta to small side dishes.

4.   Limit concentrated sweets – including high calorie foods with a low glycemic index, suchn as ice cream – to occasional treats. Reduce fruit juice to no more than one cup a day. Completely eliminate sugar-sweetened drinks.

5.   Eat a healthy type of protein at most meals, such as beans, fish, or skinless chicken.

6.   Choose foods with healthful fats, such as olive oil, nuts (almonds, walnuts, peacans), and avacados. Limit saturated fats from diary and other animal products. Completely eliminate partially hydrogenated fats (trans-fats), which are in fast food and many packaged foods.

7.   Have three meals and one or two snacks each day, and don't skip breakfast.

8.   Eat slowly and stop when full.

Glycemic Index for Diabetes Reversal

The glycemic index diet is a popular diet plan that focuses on foods with a low glycemic index, as they can help people better manage their blood sugar levels and promote weight loss. The diet is based on the notion that eating foods with a low glycemic index can help to regulate the body's blood sugar levels and reduce the risk of developing heart disease, type 2 diabetes, and other chronic illnesses.

The glycemic index diet works by limiting foods with a high glycemic index, such as white bread, white potatoes, and sugary breakfast cereals, and instead focusing on foods with a low glycemic index, such as whole grains, legumes, vegetables, and fruits. These foods are digested more slowly, which helps to keep blood sugar levels stable throughout the day and prevents blood sugar spikes and dips. Eating foods with a low glycemic index can also help you feel fuller for longer and reduce hunger cravings.

The glycemic index diet also encourages people to

include healthy fats, such as olive oil and nuts, in their diets, as well as lean proteins, such as fish, lean poultry, and legumes. Eating these foods in combination with low glycemic index foods can help to fill you up and keep you feeling full for longer, thus reducing the risk of overeating and snacking.

In addition to helping with weight loss and regulating blood sugar levels, the glycemic index diet can also help improve cholesterol levels. Eating foods with a low glycemic index can help reduce LDL cholesterol and increase HDL cholesterol, which can help lower the risk of developing heart disease.

Overall, the glycemic index diet can be a helpful tool for those looking to lose weight and improve their overall health. By focusing on foods with a low glycemic index, such as whole grains, legumes, vegetables, and fruits, and limiting foods with a high glycemic index, such as white bread, white potatoes, and sugary breakfast cereals, you can help to regulate your body's blood sugar levels, improve cholesterol levels, and reduce your risk of developing chronic conditions.

This diet is not only beneficial for weight loss, but it can also improve your overall health and well-being. Low glycemic index diet is highly recommended. The guilding principle is low Carbohydrates, low fat, moderate protein, and high mineral and vitamins.

CHAPTER 3

DIABETES REVERSAL DIET

Diabetes is a chronic condition that affects the body's ability to process glucose, or sugar, in the blood. It can lead to serious health complications if left untreated, so it is important to understand the basics of diabetes and diet.

The primary goal of managing diabetes is to keep blood sugar levels within a healthy range. This can be achieved through diet, exercise, and, if needed, medication. Eating a healthy and balanced diet is essential for controlling diabetes. Foods should be low in saturated fat and cholesterol and provide plenty of vitamins, minerals, and fiber. Eating foods that are high in fiber can help keep blood sugar levels in check and reduce the risk of complications.

It is also important to monitor carbohydrate intake. Foods high in carbohydrates can cause a spike in blood sugar, so it is important to be aware of how many carbohydrates are in each meal. It might also be beneficial to eat smaller meals more often throughout the day.

Exercising regularly can also help manage diabetes. Exercise helps to lower blood sugar levels, reduce stress, and promote weight loss.

Finally, it is important to monitor blood sugar levels and get regular check-ups with your doctor. These will help to make sure that diabetes is being managed properly and that any complications can be caught and treated early.

Overall, managing diabetes is a lifelong commitment. Eating a healthy, balanced diet, exercising regularly, and monitoring blood sugar levels are all important steps in managing diabetes. With the right lifestyle and diet, diabetes can be managed and complications can be prevented.

DIABETES REVERSAL DIET - TIP 1:

- **Choose High Fibre, Slow-release Carbs**

Carbohydrates have a big impact on your blood sugar levels more than fats and proteins, but you don't have to avoid them. You just need to be very smart on what types of carbs you eat. In general, it's best to limit highly refined carbohydrates like white bread, pasta, and rice, as well as soda, candy and snacks foods. Focus instead on high fibre complex carbohydrates - also known as slow-release carbs. Slow-release carbs help keep blood sugar levels even because they arc digested more slowly. Thus, preventing your body from producing too much insulin. They also provide lasting energy and help you stay full longer.

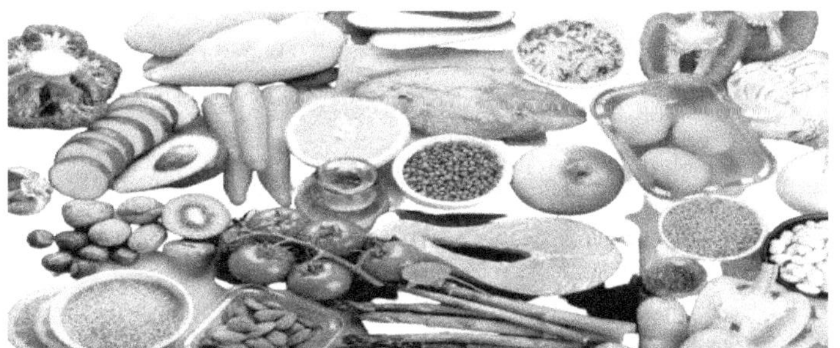

Choosing carbs that packed with fibre (and don't spike:

blood sugar)

Instead of...	Try these high fibre options...
White rice	Brown rice or wild rice
White potatoes (including fries and mashed potatoes)	Sweet potatoes, yams, squash, cauliflower mash
Regular pasta	Whole wheat pasta
White bread	Whole wheat or whole grain
Sugary breakfast cereal	High fibre breakfast cereal
Instant oakmeal	Steel-cut oats or rolled oats
Croissant or pastry	Bran muffin

DIABETES REVERSAL DIET - TIP 2:

- **Choose Fats Wisely**

Fats can be either helpful or harmful in your diet. People with diabetes are at high risk for heart disease. So it is even more important to be smart about fats. Some fats are unhealthy and others have enormous health benefits. But, all fats are high iin calories, so you should always watch your portion sizes.

Unhealthy Fats – The two most damaging fats are saturated fats and Trans-fats. Saturated fats are found mainly in animal products such as red meat, whole milk dairy products, and eggs. Trans-fats, also called partially hydrogenated oils, are created by adding hydrogen to liquid vegetable oiils to make them more solid and less likely to spoil - which is very good for food manufacturers, and very bad for you.

Healthy Fats - The best fats are unsaturated fats, which come from plant and fish sources and are liquid at room temperature. Primary sources include olive oil, canola oil, nuts, and avocados. Also focus on omega-3 fatty acids, which fight inflammation and support brain and heart health. Good sources include salmon, yuna, and flaxseeds.

Ways to Reduce Unhealthy Fats and Add Healthy Fats:

- Cook with olive oil instead of butter or vegetable oil.

- Trim any visible fat off of meat before cooking and remove the skin before cooking chicken and turkey.

- Instead of chips or crackers, try snacking on nuts or seeds. Add them to your morning cereal or have a little handful for a filling snack. Nuts butter are also very satisfying and full of healthy fats.

- Instead of frying, choose to grill, boil, bake, or stir-fry.

- Serve fish 2 or 3 times a week instead of red meat.

- Add avocado to your sandwiches instead of cheese. This will keep the creamy texture, but improve the health factor.

- When baking, use canola oil or applesauce instead of butter.

- Rather than using heavy cream, make your soups

creamy by adding low-fat milk thickened with flour, pureed potatoes, or reduced fat sour cream.

DIABETES REVERSAL DIET – TIP 3

- **Eat at Regularly Set Times**

If you're overweight, you may be encouraged to note that you only have to lose 7% of your body weight to cut your risk of diabetes in half. And you don't have to obsessively count calories or starve yourself to do it. Your body is better able to regulate blood sugar levels and your weight, when you maintain a regular meal schedule. Aim for moderate and consistent portion sizes for each meal or snack.

- **Don't skip breakfast.** Start your day off with a good breakfast. Eating breakfast everyday will help you have energy as well as steady blood sugar levels.

- **Eat regular small meals – up to 6 per day.** People tend to eat larger portions when they are overly hungry, so eating regularly will help you keep your portions in check.

- **Keep calorie intake the same.** Regulating

the amount of calories you eat on a day-to-day basis has an impact on the regularity of your blood sugar levels. Try to eat roughly the same amount of calories everyday, rather than over eating one day or at one meal and then skimping on the next.

DIABETES REVERSAL DIET – TIP 4

- **Keep a Food Diary**

Research shows that people who keep a food diary are more likely to lose weight and keep it off. In fact, a recent study found out that people who kept food diary lost twice as much weight as those who didn't. Why does wring down what you ear and drink help you drop pounds? For me, it helps you identify problem areas – such as your afternoon snack or your morning latte – where you're getting a lot more calories than you realized. It also increases your awareness of what, why, and how much you're eating helps you cut back on mindless snacking and emotional eating.

By following a healthy glycemic diet, people with

diabetes can better manage their condition and improve their overall health. Keeping a food diary is a great way to help control diabetes. It provides a way to track and monitor what you are eating when you are eating it, and how much you are eating. By tracking your food intake, you can better adjust your diet to help manage your blood sugar levels. You can also use the diary to identify triggers that can increase your risk of diabetes and identify unhealthy eating patterns. With a food diary, you have a better understanding of your food choices and can make better decisions to help you manage your diabetes.

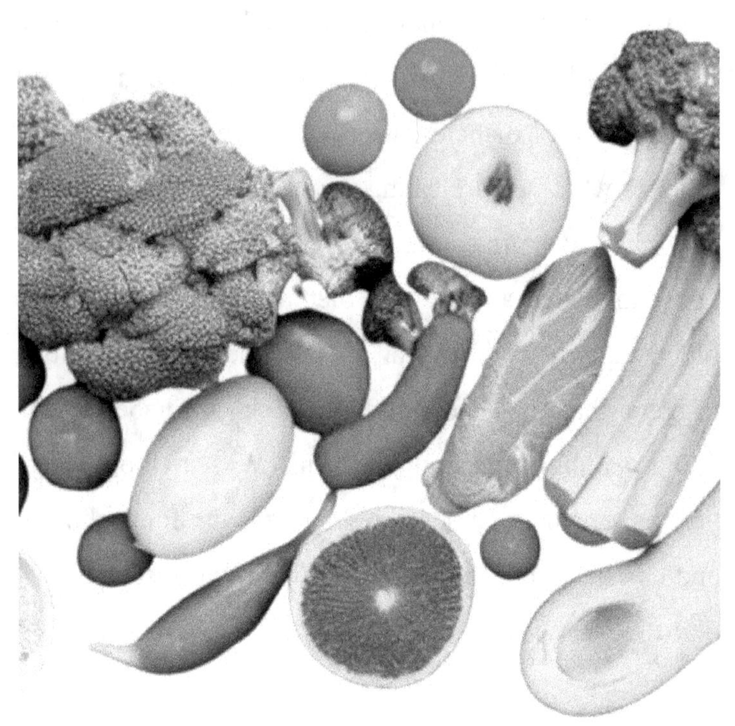

CHAPTER 4

ADDITIONAL TIPS FOR DIABETES REVERSAL AND DIET

Vitamins and Supplements

Research has shown that vitamin supplements have no benefit for heart disease and diabetes. Because of the lack of scientific evidence for benefit, the American Diabetes Association does not recommend regular use of vitamin supplements, except for people who have vitamin deficiencies. Parents with type 2 diabetes who take metformin (Glucophage) should be aware that this drug can interfere with vitamins B12 absorption. Calcium supplements may help counteract metformin – associated vitamin B12 deficiency.

Sodium (Salt)

It is important for everyone to restrict their sodium (salt) intake. People with diabetes should reduce sodium intake to less than 1500mgdaily. Limiting or avoiding consumption of processed foods can go a long way to reducing salt intake. Simply eliminating table and cooking salt is also beneficial. Salt substitutes, such as Nusalt and Mrs. Dash (which contain mixtures of potassium, sodium, and magnesium) are available, but they can be risky for people with kidney disease or those who take blood pressure medication that causes potassium retention. Similarly, while eating more potassium rich foods is helpful for achieving healthy blood pressure, patients with diabetes should check with their doctors before increasing the amount of potassium in their diets.

OTHER MINERALS

Calcium – Calcium supplements may be important in older patients with diabetes to help reduce the risk for osteoporosis, particularly if their diets are low in diary products.

Magnesium – Magnesium deficiency may have some role in insulin resistance and high blood pressure.

Research indicates that magnesium rich diets may help lower type 2 diabetes risk. Whole grain breads and cereals, nuts (such as spinach, avocados, and beans) are excellent dietary sources of magnesium. Dietary supplements do not provide any benefit. Persons who live in soft water areas, who use diuretics, or who have other risk factors for magnesium deficiency may require more dietary magnesium than others.

Selenium – Selenium, a trace mineral, may increase diabetes risk. An average healthy diet supplies adequate amounts of selenium. There is no need to take dietary supplements.

EXCERCISE

When it comes to preventing, controlling, or reversing diabetes, you can't afford to overlook exercise. Exercise can help your weight loss efforts, and is especially important in maintaining weight loss. There is also evidence that regular exercise can improve your insulin sensitivity even if you don't loss weight.

Exercise is an essential part of managing diabetes, and it can have a range of positive effects on the health of a diabetic patient. Exercise can help to regulate blood sugar levels, improve circulation, and reduce the risk of diabetes-related complications. It can also help to reduce the risk of cardiovascular disease, improve mental health, and promote weight loss.

One of the primary benefits of exercise for a diabetic patient is its ability to regulate blood sugar levels. Exercise helps to reduce glucose levels in the blood by increasing the body's sensitivity to insulin, which is the hormone responsible for regulating blood sugar. Regular exercise can also help to prevent the onset of type-2 diabetes, by making the body more efficient at using insulin.

Exercise can also help to improve circulation, which is important for a diabetic patient. Poor circulation can lead to complications such as diabetic neuropathy, which is a type of nerve damage that can occur due to poor circulation. Exercise can help to improve circulation by promoting the flow of oxygen and nutrients to the cells. This helps to reduce the risk of complications associated with diabetes, such as stroke and heart attack.

Exercise can also help to reduce the risk of cardiovascular disease, which is a common complication of diabetes. Regular exercise helps to reduce the risk of heart disease and stroke by improving blood pressure and cholesterol levels. Exercise can also help to reduce the risk of obesity, which is a major risk factor for developing type-2 diabetes.

Finally, exercise can help to improve mental health and reduce stress levels. Diabetes can be a stressful condition, and regular exercise can help to reduce stress and improve mood. Exercise has also been shown to improve sleep quality and reduce fatigue, which can help to improve overall health and well-being.

In conclusion, exercise is an important part of managing diabetes and has a range of benefits for diabetic patients.

Regular exercise can help to regulate blood sugar levels, improve circulation, reduce the risk of cardiovascular disease, improve mental health, and promote weight loss. For these reasons, exercise should be an essential part of any diabetic patient's care plan. You don't have to become a gym rat or adopt a grueling fitness regimen. One of the easiest ways is to start walking for 30minutes five or more times a week. You can also try swimming, biking, or any other moderate intensity activities – meaning you work up a light sweat and start to breathe harder.

If your last diet attempt wasn't successful, or life events have caused you to gain weight, don't be discouraged. The key is to find a plan that works with your body's individual needs so that you can avoid common diet pitfalls and instead make lasting lifestyle changes that can help you find long term weight loss success.

CHAPTER 5

LOW GLYCEMIC INDEX MEAL PLAN FOR DIABETES REVERSAL

DAY 1

BREAKFAST: Overnight oats with chia seeds, ground flaxseed, and almond milk

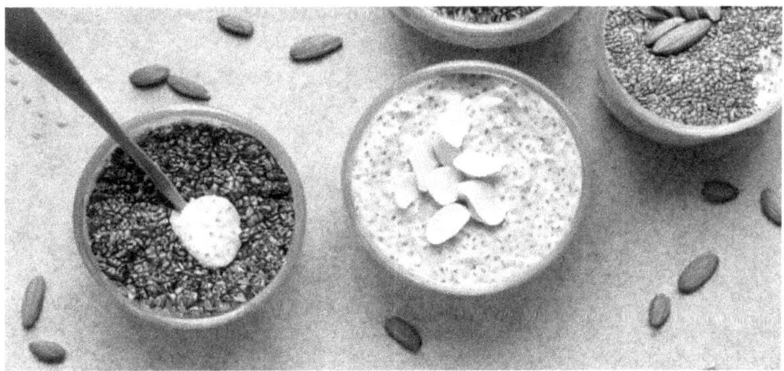

Prep Time: 5 minutes

Calorie Count: 370

GI Range: Low

Ingredients:

- ½ cup rolled oats

- 2 tablespoons chia seeds

- 2 tablespoons ground flaxseed

- 1 cup almond milk

- 1 tablespoon honey

Preparation Instructions:

1. Combine the oats, chia seeds, ground flaxseed, almond milk, and honey in a bowl or Mason jar.

2. Stir until everything is mixed together.

3. Cover with a lid or plastic wrap and refrigerate overnight.

4. In the morning, stir the oats and enjoy!

SNACK: Celery sticks with almond Butter

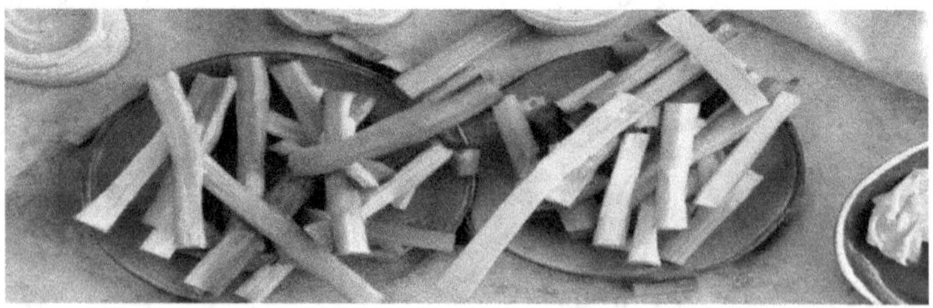

Prep Time: 10 minutes

GI Range: Low

Calorie Count: 100 Calories

Ingredients:

- 2 celery stalks

- 2 tablespoons almond butter

Preparation Instructions:

1. Wash and dry the celery stalks.

2. Cut the celery stalks into 3-4 inch pieces.

3. Spread the almond butter evenly over the celery pieces.

4. Enjoy!

LUNCH: Quinoa and black bean salad with olive oil, lemon juice, and fresh herbs

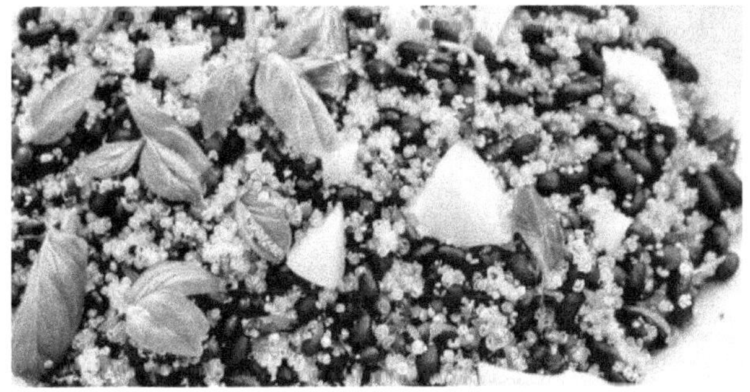

Prep Time: 10 minutes

GI Range: Low

Calorie Count: 303 per serving

Ingredients:

- 1 cup quinoa

- 1 can black beans, rinsed and drained

- ½ cup olive oil

- 3 tablespoons fresh lemon juice

- 2 tablespoons fresh oregano, chopped

- 1 teaspoon sea salt

- ½ teaspoon ground black pepper

- ½ cup fresh parsley, chopped

- 2 tablespoons fresh thyme, chopped

Preparation Instructions:

1. Cook quinoa according to package instructions.

2. Meanwhile, in a large bowl, combine black beans, olive oil, lemon juice, oregano, salt, and pepper.

3. Add cooked quinoa and mix until all ingredients are evenly distributed.

4. Fold in parsley and thyme until just combined.

5. Serve immediately or chill in the refrigerator for up to eight hours. Enjoy!

SNACK: Apple slices with natural peanut butter

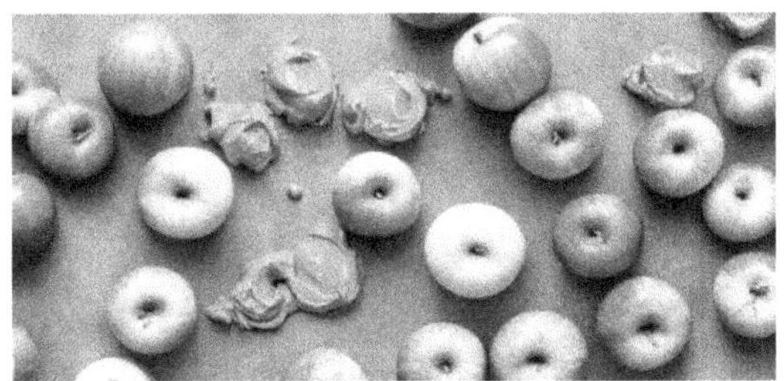

Prep Time: 5 minutes

GI Range: Low

Calorie Count: 150

Ingredients:

- 2 apples, cored and thinly sliced

- 2 tablespoons natural peanut butter

- 2 tablespoons chopped walnuts (optional)

- 1 tablespoon honey (optional)

Preparation Instructions:

1. On a platter, arrange the apple slices.

2. Spread the natural peanut butter over the apple slices.

3. Sprinkle the chopped walnuts and honey over the peanut butter (optional).

4. Serve and enjoy!

DINNER: Grilled salmon with roasted asparagus

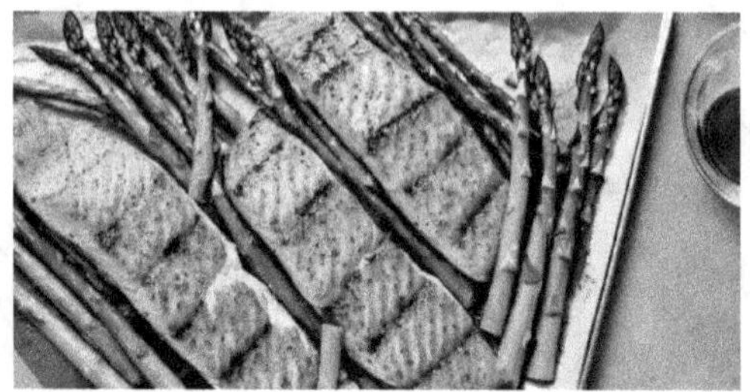

Prep Time: 15 minutes

GI Range: Low

Calorie Count: 533

Ingredients:

-4 salmon fillets

-1 teaspoon olive oil

-1 teaspoon smoked paprika

-1/2 teaspoon garlic powder

-1/4 teaspoon ground black pepper

-1/4 teaspoon sea salt

-1 pound fresh asparagus, trimmed

-1 tablespoon olive oil

-1/4 teaspoon sea salt

Preparation Instructions:

1. Preheat the grill to medium-high heat.

2. In a small bowl, combine the olive oil, smoked paprika, garlic powder, black pepper, and salt. Rub the mixture on both sides of the salmon fillets.

3. Place the salmon fillets on the preheated grill. Cook the salmon for 4–5 minutes on each side, or until it is done.

4. Meanwhile, preheat the oven to 425°F.

5. Place the asparagus on a baking sheet. Salt and olive oil are drizzled on top. To coat, toss.

6. Roast the asparagus in the preheated oven for 10–12 minutes, or until tender.

7. Serve the grilled salmon with the roasted asparagus. Enjoy!

DAY 2

BREAKFAST: Scrambled eggs with spinach and tomatoes

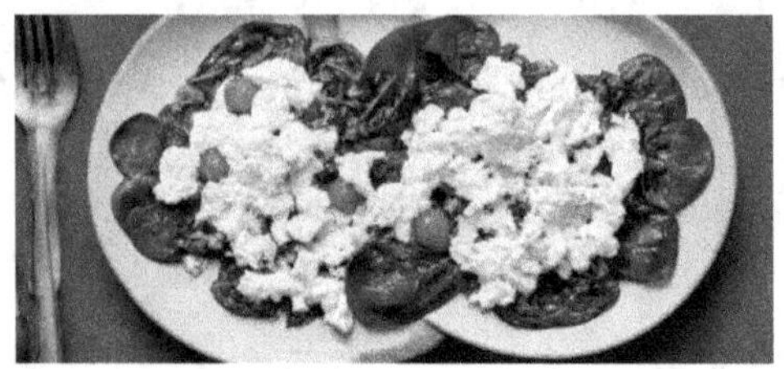

Prep Time: 10 minutes

GI Range: Low

Calorie Count: 170 calories

Ingredients:

- 2 eggs

- 2 tablespoons of milk

- 2 tablespoons of olive oil

- 1 cup of spinach

- 1/2 cup of cherry tomatoes, quartered

- Salt and pepper to taste

Preparation Instructions:

1. Heat the olive oil in a medium-sized skillet over medium heat.

2. Add the spinach and tomatoes to the skillet and cook until the spinach is wilted and the tomatoes are soft

about 3-4 minutes.

3. In a medium bowl, whisk together the eggs, milk, salt, and pepper until combined.

4. Pour the egg mixture into the skillet and cook, occasionally stirring, until the eggs are cooked, about 5 minutes.

5. Serve the scrambled eggs with spinach and tomatoes warm. Enjoy!

SNACK: Greek yogurt with fresh berries

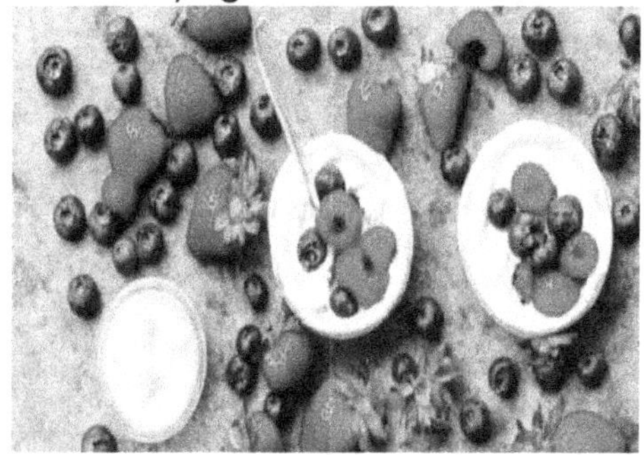

Prep Time: 5 minutes

GI Range: Low

Calorie Count: 200-250 calories

Ingredients:

  -1 cup plain Greek yogurt

  -1/4 cup fresh blueberries

  -1/4 cup fresh raspberries

-1/4 cup fresh strawberries

-1-2 tablespoons honey

Preparation Instructions:

1. In a medium bowl, combine the Greek yogurt and honey.

2. Add in the fresh berries and mix gently.

3. Divide the yogurt and berry mixture into two bowls.

4. Enjoy!

LUNCH: Kale and white bean soup

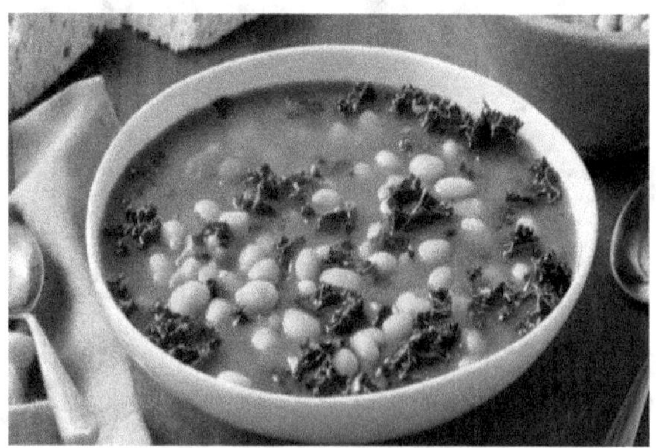

Prep Time: 20 minutes

GI Range: Low

Calorie Count: 200 calories per serving

Ingredients:

- 2 tablespoons of extra-virgin olive oil

- 1 large onion, diced

- 2 cloves of garlic, minced

- 2 cups of vegetable broth

- Two (15-ounce) cans of washed and drained cannellini beans

- 1 bunch kale (leaves and stems removed).

- 1 teaspoon of dried oregano

- 1 teaspoon of dried basil

- Salt and pepper, to taste

Preparation Instructions:

1. Over medium heat, warm the olive oil in a big saucepan.

2. Add the onion and garlic, and sauté for about 5 minutes, until the onion is softened.

3. Pour in the vegetable broth and add the cannellini beans. Boil for a few minutes, then turn down the heat and simmer for approximately ten minutes.

4. Add the kale and season with oregano, basil, salt, and pepper. Simmer for an additional 5 minutes, until the kale is softened.

5. Serve the soup hot with a sprinkle of Parmesan cheese, if desired. Enjoy!

SNACK: Carrot and celery sticks with hummus

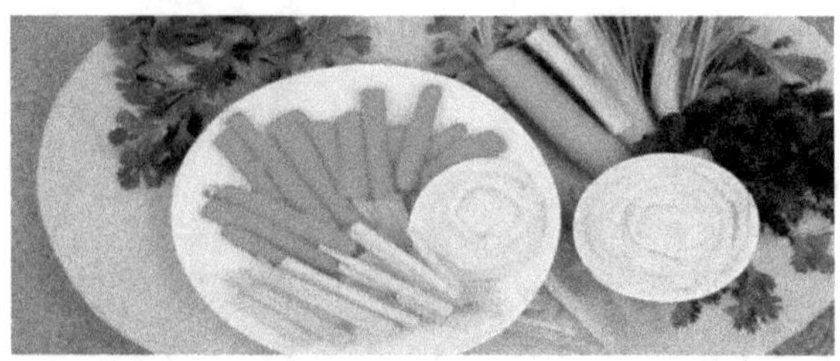

Prep Time: 10 minutes

GI Range: Low

Calorie Count: 83 calories per serving

Ingredients:

- 2 large carrots, peeled and cut into sticks

- 2 large stalks of celery cut into sticks

- 1 cup of hummus

Preparation Instructions:

1. Begin by peeling and cutting 2 large carrots into sticks.

2. Cut 2 large stalks of celery into sticks.

3. Place the carrot and celery sticks on a plate.

4. Spoon 1 cup of hummus onto the plate and spread it evenly over the vegetables.

5. Serve the carrot and celery sticks with hummus and enjoy!

DINNER: Grilled chicken with roasted vegetables

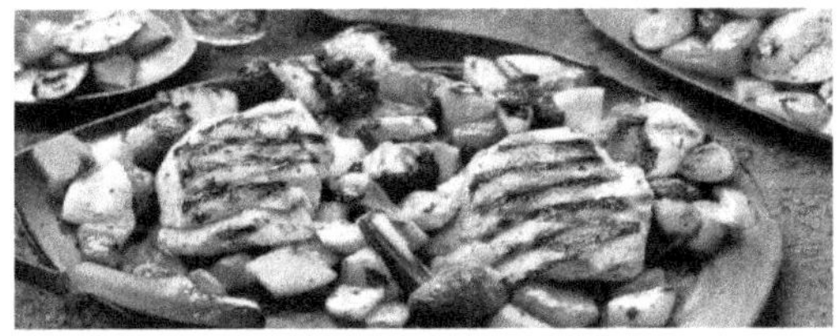

Prep Time: 45 minutes

GI Range: Low

Calorie Count: 464 calories

Ingredients:

- 2 boneless, skinless chicken breasts

- 1 red bell pepper, diced

- 1 yellow bell pepper, diced

- 1 zucchini, diced

- 1 red onion, diced

- 2 tablespoons olive oil

- Salt and pepper, to taste

- 1 teaspoon garlic powder

- 1 teaspoon smoked paprika

Preparation Instructions:

1. Preheat the grill to medium-high heat.

2. Place chicken breasts in a shallow dish and season

with salt, pepper, garlic powder, and smoked paprika.

3. In a bowl, combine the diced red bell pepper, yellow bell pepper, zucchini, red onion, and olive oil. To taste, add salt and pepper to the dish.

4. Grill the chicken breasts for 4-5 minutes per side, or until cooked through.

5. Meanwhile, place the vegetables on the grill and cook for 5-7 minutes, or until tender and lightly charred.

6. Serve the grilled chicken with the roasted vegetables. Enjoy!

DAY 3

BREAKFAST: Oatmeal with chopped walnuts and almond milk

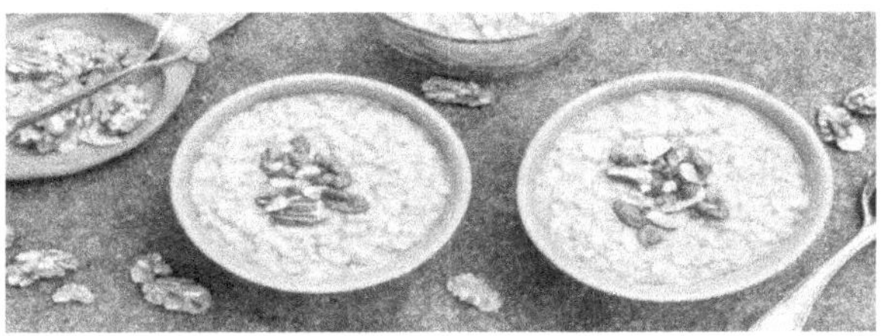

Prep Time: 5 minutes

GI Range: Low

Calorie Count: 320

Ingredients:

- 1 cup of rolled oats

- 2 cups of almond milk

- 2 tablespoons of chopped walnuts

- Cinnamon, to taste

- One teaspoonful of honey or maple syrup (optional)

Preparation Instructions:

1. Pour the rolled oats into a medium-sized saucepan.

2. Pour the almond milk into the saucepan and turn the heat to medium.

3. Stir the oats and almond milk together until they are

combined.

4. Allow the oatmeal to cook for about 4–5 minutes, stirring occasionally.

5. Once the oatmeal is cooked, remove it from the heat and add the chopped walnuts, cinnamon, and honey or maple syrup (if desired).

6. Stir the ingredients together until combined.

7. Serve the oatmeal warm and enjoy!

SNACK: Air-popped popcorn

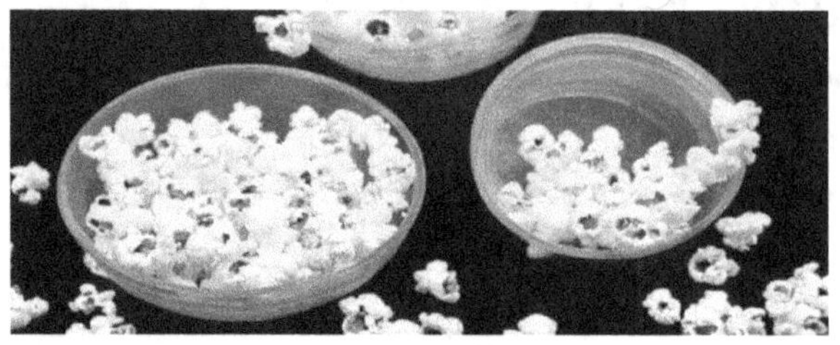

Prep Time: 5 minutes

GI Range: Low

Calories: 30 calories per cup

Ingredients:

-1/4 cup of popcorn kernels

-1 tablespoon of vegetable oil

-Salt to taste (optional)

Preparation Instructions:

1. Put the oil and the popcorn kernels in a large pot, and put it on the stove over medium heat.

2. Shake the pot periodically, so that all of the kernels are coated with the oil and are heated evenly.

3. Once the popping has slowed to several seconds between each pop, remove the pot from the heat and pour the popcorn into a bowl.

4. Sprinkle with salt to taste, if desired.

5. Enjoy!

LUNCH: Lentil and quinoa salad with olive oil and lemon juice

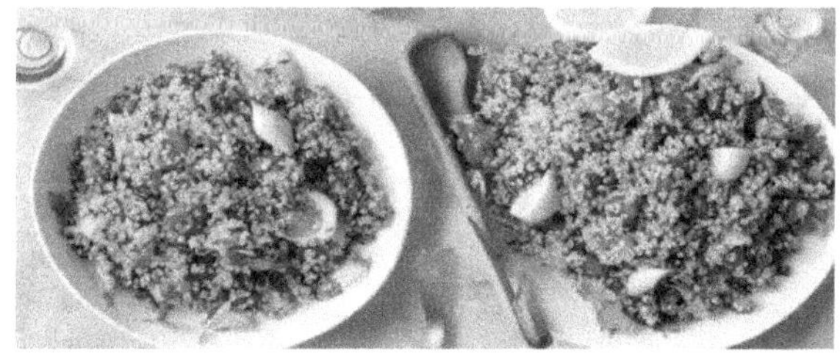

Prep Time: 10 minutes

GI Range: Low

Calorie Count: 257 calories

Ingredients:

- 1 cup cooked lentils

- 1 cup cooked quinoa

- 1/4 cup sliced olives

- 1/4 cup diced red onion

- 2 tablespoons olive oil

- 2 tablespoons lemon juice

- 1 teaspoon Dijon mustard

- Salt and pepper to taste

Preparation Instructions:

1. In a large bowl, combine the cooked lentils, quinoa, olives, and red onion.

2. In a separate bowl, whisk together the olive oil, lemon juice, and Dijon mustard. To check, add salt and pepper to the food.

3. Pour the dressing over the lentil and quinoa mixture and mix until everything is evenly coated.

4. Serve the salad at room temperature or chilled. Enjoy!

SNACK: Cucumber slices with cottage cheese

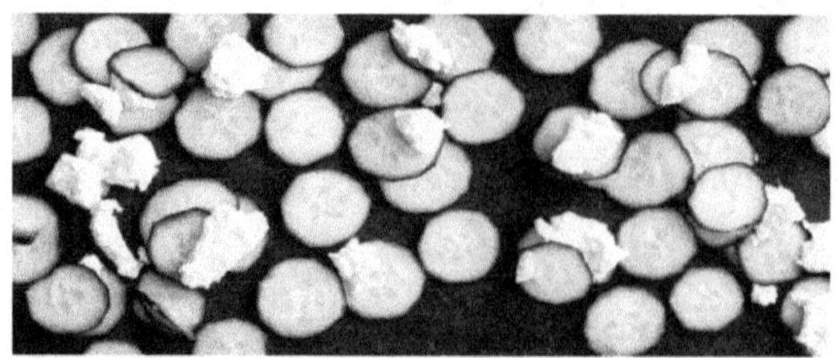

Prep Time: 10 minutes

GI Range: Low-Medium

Calorie Count: Approximately 60 calories per serving

Ingredients:

-1 cucumber, thinly sliced

-1/2 cup cottage cheese

-1/4 teaspoon garlic powder

-1/4 teaspoon onion powder

-1/4 teaspoon parsley

-1/4 teaspoon dill

-1/4 teaspoon black pepper

Preparation Instructions:

1. Set the oven's temperature to 375°F.

2. Slice the cucumber into thin slices and arrange them on a baking sheet.

3. Sprinkle garlic powder, onion powder, parsley, dill, and black pepper over the cucumber slices.

4. Bake the cucumbers for 10 minutes.

5. Meanwhile, combine the cottage cheese with the seasonings in a small bowl.

6. Remove the cucumbers from the oven, and let them cool for a few minutes.

7. Top each cucumber slice with a spoonful of the

cottage cheese mixture.

8. Serve the cucumber slices with cottage cheese immediately. Enjoy!

DINNER: Baked salmon with brown rice and steamed vegetables

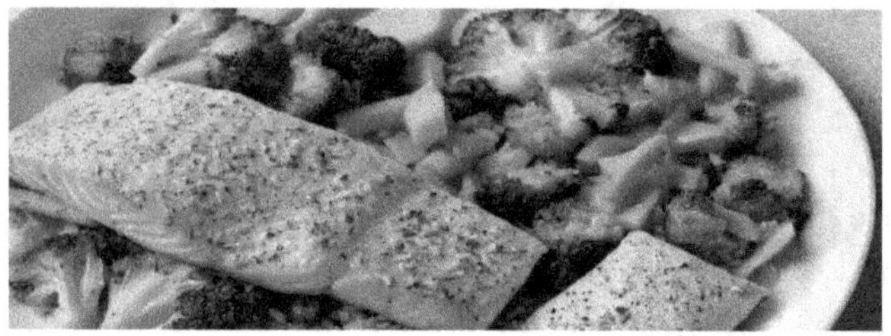

Prep Time: 15 minutes

GI Range: Low

Calorie Count: 332 Calories

Ingredients:

- 4 (6-oz) salmon fillets

- 2 tablespoons olive oil, divided

- 1 teaspoon garlic powder

- Salt and freshly ground black pepper

- 1 cup brown rice

- 2 cups vegetable stock

- 1/2 cup frozen peas

- 1/2 cup diced carrots

- 1/2 cup diced red bell pepper

- 2 tablespoons chopped fresh parsley

Preparation Instructions:

1. Preheat oven to 425°F.

2. Line a baking sheet with parchment paper and brush with 1 tablespoon of olive oil.

3. Place the salmon fillets on the parchment paper and season with garlic powder, salt, and pepper. Drizzle with the remaining 1 tablespoon of olive oil.

4. Bake the salmon for 10-12 minutes, or until cooked through.

5. Meanwhile, cook the brown rice according to package instructions, using the vegetable stock in place of water.

6. Once the rice is cooked, add the peas, carrots, bell pepper, and parsley to the pot and stir to combine.

7. Serve the salmon over the rice and vegetables and enjoy!

DAY 4

BREAKFAST: Banana, almond milk, and spinach smoothie

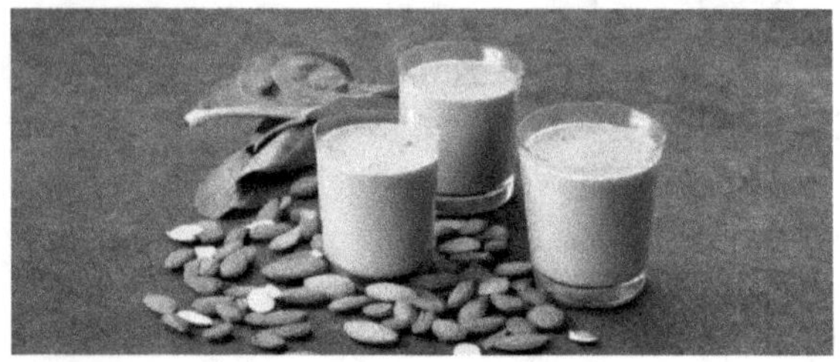

Prep Time: 10 minutes

GI range: Low

Calorie Count: 220

Ingredients:

- 2 ripe bananas
- 1 cup almond milk
- 1 cup spinach
- 2 tablespoons raw honey
- 1 teaspoon vanilla extract
- 1/2 cup ice

Preparation Instructions:

1. Peel and slice the bananas.

2. Place all ingredients in a blender.

3. Blend on high until smooth.

4. Serve cold.

SNACK: Almonds

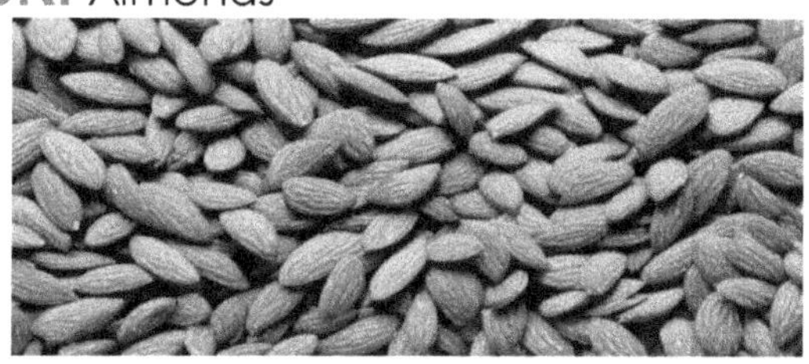

Prep Time: 10 minutes

GI Range: Low

Calorie Count: 160 calories per 1/4 cup

Ingredients:

-1/4 cup blanched almonds

-1 tablespoon olive oil

-1/4 teaspoon salt

Preparation Instructions:

1. Preheat the oven to 350°F.

2. On a baking sheet, spread the blanched almonds out.

3. Drizzle the olive oil over the almonds and sprinkle with salt.

4. Bake for 10 minutes, stirring occasionally to ensure they are evenly cooked. Allow the almonds to cool before serving.

LUNCH: Vegetable stir-fry with brown rice and tofu

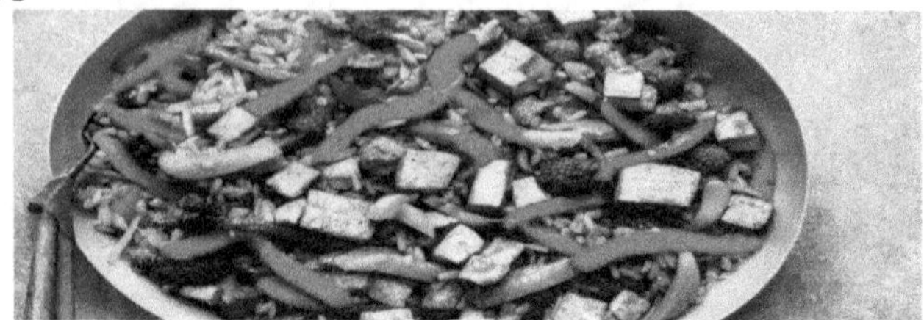

Prep Time: 15 minutes

GI Range: 45-55

Calorie Count: 495 calories

Ingredients:

- 1 cup uncooked brown rice

- 1/2 cup vegetable broth

- 1 tablespoon sesame oil

- 1/2 cup diced onion

- 1/2 cup diced bell peppers

- 1/2 cup sliced mushrooms

- 1/2 cup diced carrots

- 1/2 cup diced zucchini

- 1 cup diced firm tofu

- 2 tablespoons soy sauce

- 1 tablespoon honey

- 1 teaspoon garlic powder

- 1 teaspoon ground ginger

Preparation Instructions:

1. Begin by cooking the brown rice according to the package instructions, using the vegetable broth instead of water.

2. In a large skillet over medium-high heat, warm the sesame oil.

3. Add the diced onion, bell peppers, mushrooms, carrots, and zucchini. Cook for 5 minutes, stirring occasionally.

4. Add the diced tofu and cook for an additional 3 minutes.

5. In a small bowl, combine the soy sauce, honey, garlic powder, and ground ginger.

6. Pour the mixture into the skillet and stir to coat all of the vegetables and tofu.

7. Cook for an additional 3 minutes, stirring occasionally.

8. Serve the stir-fry over the cooked brown rice. Enjoy!

SNACK: Celery sticks with almond butter

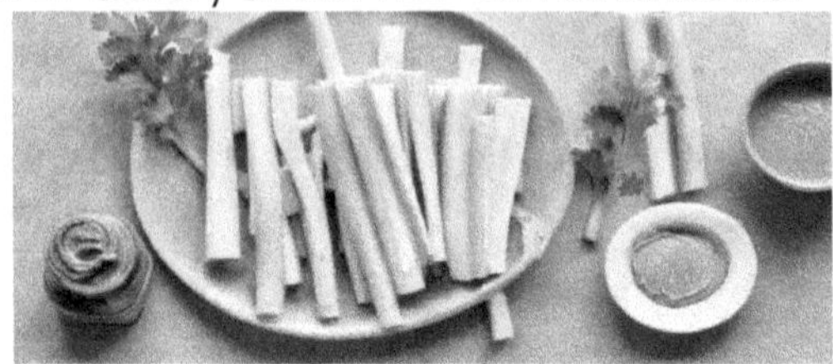

Prep Time: 10 minutes

GI range: Low

Calorie Count: Approximately 125 calories

Ingredients:

-2 celery stalks

-2 tablespoons of almond butter

Preparation Instructions:

1. Wash the celery stalks and pat dry with a paper towel.

2. Cut the celery stalks into sticks and set them aside.

3. Place the almond butter in a bowl and microwave for 10-20 seconds, or until it has softened.

4. Dip the celery sticks into the almond butter and enjoy!

DINNER: Grilled chicken with roasted sweet potatoes

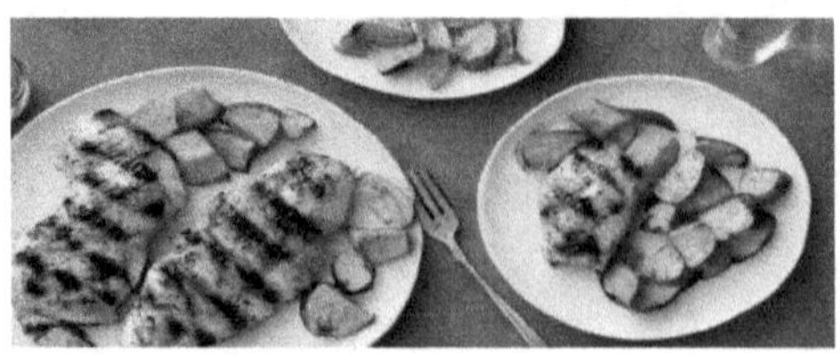

Prep Time: 15 minutes

Cook Time: 25 minutes

Total Time: 40 minutes

GI Range: Low

Calorie Count: 270 calories per serving

Ingredients:

-2 boneless, skinless chicken breasts

-1 teaspoon garlic powder

-1 teaspoon onion powder

-1 teaspoon paprika

-1 teaspoon chili powder

-1/2 teaspoon ground cumin

-1/2 teaspoon black pepper

-1/4 teaspoon cayenne pepper (optional)

-1 tablespoon olive oil

-2 sweet potatoes, cubed

-Salt and pepper, to taste

Preparation Instructions:

1. Preheat the oven to 400°F and lightly grease a baking sheet.

2. In a small bowl, mix together the garlic powder, onion powder, paprika, chili powder, cumin, black

pepper, and cayenne pepper.

3. Rub the spice mixture onto the chicken breasts and set aside.

4. Place the sweet potatoes on the greased baking sheet. Sprinkle with pepper and salt and drizzle with olive oil. Toss to combine.

5. Place the chicken breasts on the baking sheet, making sure not to overlap them with the sweet potatoes.

6. Bake in the preheated oven for 25 minutes, or until the chicken is cooked through and the potatoes are tender.

7. Heat a grill pan over medium-high heat. Add the chicken breasts and cook for 3–4 minutes per side, or until lightly charred and cooked through.

8. Serve the grilled chicken with the roasted sweet potatoes. Enjoy!

DAY 5

BREAKFAST: Avocado toast with poached eggs

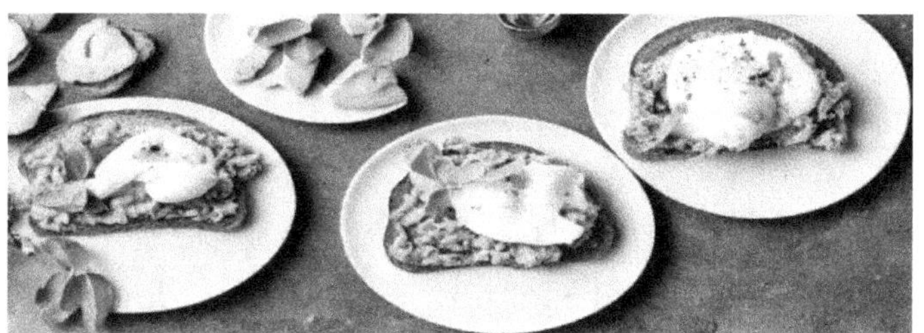

Prep Time: 10 minutes

GI Range: Low

Calorie Count: 530

Ingredients:

- 2 slices of multigrain bread
- 2 eggs
- 2 tsp of white vinegar
- 2 ripe avocados
- 2 tbsp of olive oil
- Salt and pepper to taste

Preparation instructions:

1. Bring a medium saucepan of water to a boil and add the white vinegar.

2. Reduce the heat and gently crack the eggs into the water. Give the eggs three to four minutes to cook.

3. Meanwhile, toast the bread.

4. After the eggs are done cooking, remove them from the water and set aside.

5. Peel the avocados and mash them in a bowl until creamy.

6. Spread the mashed avocado onto the toast slices.

7. Place the poached eggs on top of the avocado toast.

8. Drizzle the olive oil over the eggs and season with salt and pepper. Serve and enjoy!

SNACK: Apple slices with natural peanut butter

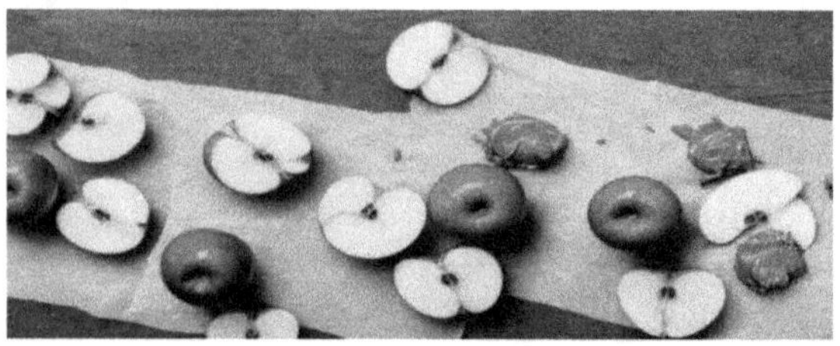

Prep Time: 5 minutes

GI Range: Low

Calorie Count: Approximately 158 (per serving)

Ingredients:

- 2 Apples

- 2 tablespoons Natural Peanut Butter

Preparation Instructions:

1. Slice apples into thin slices.

2. Spread natural peanut butter over each slice.

3. Enjoy your snack!

LUNCH: Roasted vegetable quinoa bowl

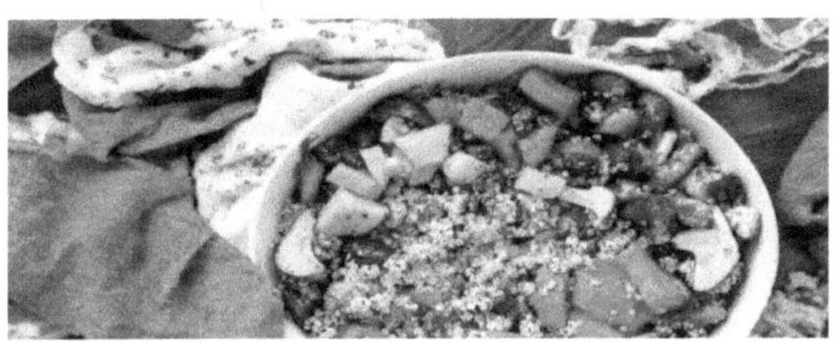

Prep Time: 10 minutes

GI Range: Low

Calories: 431

Ingredients:

- 2 Medium-sized zucchinis

- 2 Medium-sized sweet potatoes

- 2 Tablespoons olive oil

- 1/2 Teaspoon garlic powder

- 1/2 Teaspoon paprika

- 1/4 Teaspoon black pepper

- 1 Teaspoon sea salt

- 1 Cup quinoa

- 2 Cups vegetable broth

- 1/4 Cup diced red onion

- 1/4 Cup diced bell pepper

- 1/4 Cup diced mushrooms

- 1 Tablespoon fresh parsley

- 2 Tablespoons fresh lemon juice

- 2 Tablespoons freshly grated Parmesan cheese

Preparation Instructions:

1. Preheat the oven to 400 °F.

2. Cut the zucchini and sweet potatoes into cubes and place them on a baking sheet.

3. Drizzle with olive oil, garlic powder, paprika, black pepper, and sea salt. Toss to combine.

4. Vegetables should be roasted in the oven for 15 to 20 minutes, or until they are soft.

5. While the vegetables are roasting, rinse the quinoa in a fine mesh strainer.

6. In a medium saucepan, bring the vegetable broth to a boil. Turn down the heat to low before adding the quinoa. Simmer, and covered, for 15 minutes.

7. Once the vegetables are done roasting, remove them from the oven and set them aside.

8. In a large bowl, combine the cooked quinoa, roasted

vegetables, diced red onion, diced bell pepper, diced mushrooms, fresh parsley, fresh lemon juice, and Parmesan cheese.

9. Serve warm and enjoy!

SNACK: Whole wheat crackers with hummus

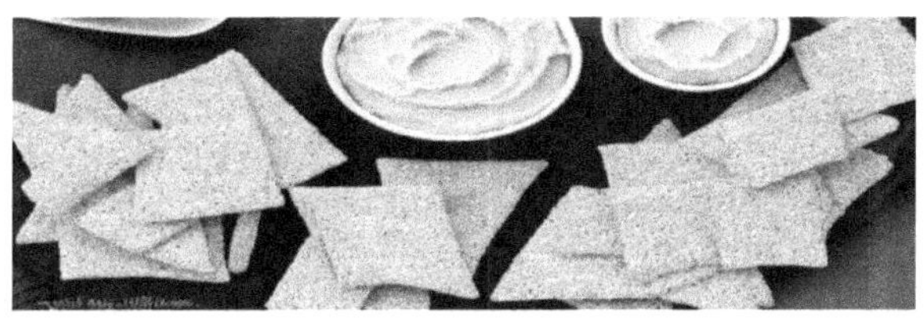

Prep Time: 15 minutes

GI Range: Low

Calorie Count: Approximately 200 per serving

Ingredients:

 -1 cup whole wheat flour

 -1/4 cup olive oil

 -1/2 teaspoon salt

 -1/2 teaspoon garlic powder

 -1/2 teaspoon onion powder

 -1/4 teaspoon black pepper

 -1/4 cup cold water

For the hummus:

 -1 can chickpeas, drained and rinsed

-2 tablespoons tahini

-1/4 cup olive oil

-1/4 cup lemon juice

-1 tablespoon garlic, minced

-1/2 teaspoon cumin

-Salt and pepper, to taste

Preparation Instructions:

1. Preheat the oven to 375°F.

2. In a medium bowl, mix together the flour, olive oil, salt, garlic powder, onion powder,, and black pepper. When dough starts to form, add the cold water and stir.

3. Turn the dough out onto a lightly floured work surface and knead for about 1 minute.

4. The dough should be rolled out to 1/8 inch thickness. Cut out crackers with a biscuit cutter or knife. Place the crackers on a baking sheet lined with parchment paper.

5. until golden brown, bake for 10 to 12 minutes.

6. For the hummus, place all ingredients in a food processor or blender and blend until smooth.

7. Serve the crackers with the hummus. Enjoy!

DINNER: Grilled salmon with roasted Brussels

sprouts

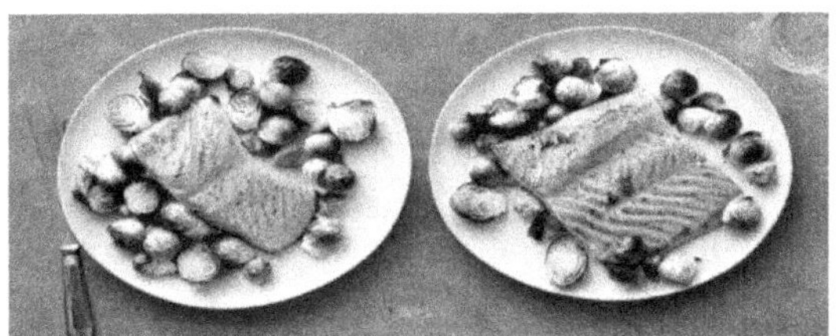

Prep Time: 15 minutes

GI Range: Low

Calorie Count: 390

Ingredients:

- 2 salmon fillets

- 1 tablespoon olive oil

- 1 teaspoon minced garlic

- 1/2 teaspoon dried oregano

- 1/4 teaspoon salt

- 1/4 teaspoon black pepper

- 12 ounces of halved and trimmed Brussels sprouts

- 1 tablespoon olive oil

- 1/4 teaspoon salt

- 1/4 teaspoon black pepper

Preparation Instructions:

1. Set the oven to 400 °F.

2. Salmon fillets should be put on a baking sheet.

Drizzle with olive oil, garlic, oregano, salt, and pepper.

3. Place the Brussels sprouts on a separate baking sheet. Sprinkle with salt, pepper, and olive oil.

4. Place both baking sheets in the preheated oven. Bake the salmon for 10 minutes and the Brussels sprout for 15 minutes, or until they are tender.

5. A grill or grill pan should be heated to medium.

6. Grill the salmon for 2 minutes per side, or until it is cooked through.

7. Serve the salmon with the roasted Brussels sprouts. Enjoy!

DAY 6

BREAKFAST: Overnight oats with chia seeds, ground flaxseed, and almond milk

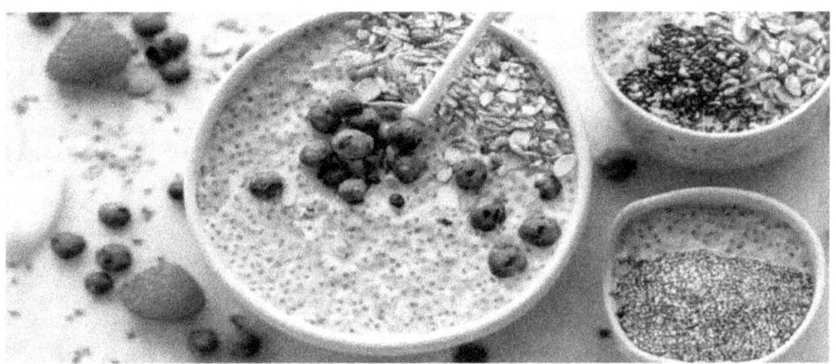

Prep Time: 10 minutes

GI Range: Low

Calorie Count: 400

Ingredients:

- -1/2 cup rolled oats
- -1/3 cup almond milk
- -1 tbsp chia seeds
- -1/2 tsp ground flaxseed
- -1 tsp maple syrup
- -1/2 banana, sliced

Preparation Instructions:

1. In a medium-sized bowl, combine the oats, chia seeds, and ground flaxseed.

2. Pour in the almond milk and whisk together until everything is well-combined.

3. Place the mixture in the refrigerator and let it sit overnight.

4. In the morning, remove the oats from the refrigerator and stir in the maple syrup.

5. Top the oats with the sliced banana.

6. Serve and enjoy!

SNACK: Greek yogurt with fresh berries

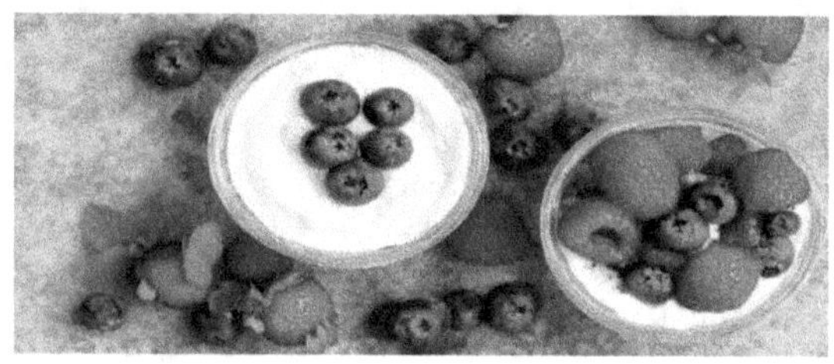

Prep time: 10 minutes

GI range: Low

Calorie count: 350

Ingredients:

-1 cup of Greek yogurt

-1/2 cup of mixed fresh berries

-1 tablespoon of honey

-1 tablespoon of slivered almonds

Preparation instructions:

1. In a medium bowl, combine the Greek yogurt and honey and mix until fully combined.

2. Add the mixed berries to the bowl and gently stir until the berries are evenly distributed throughout the yogurt.

3. Transfer the mixture to 2 serving bowls.

4. Top the yogurt with the slivered almonds.

5. Serve and enjoy!

LUNCH: Lentil and quinoa salad with olive oil and lemon juice

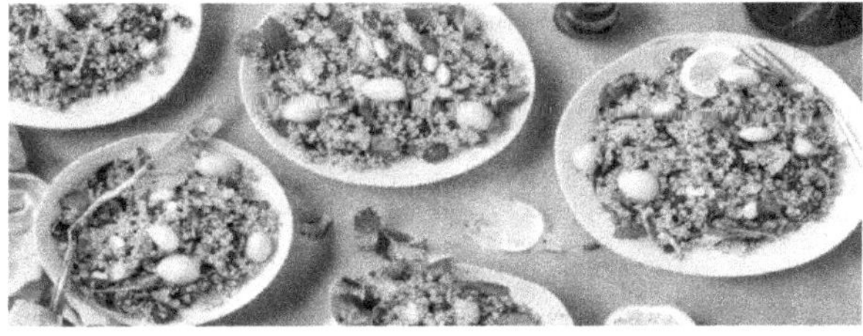

Prep Time: 20 minutes

GI Range: Low

Calorie Count: Approximately 400 calories per serving

Ingredients:

- 1 cup cooked lentils

- 1 cup cooked quinoa

- 1/4 cup chopped red onion

- 1/4 cup chopped red bell pepper

- 1/4 cup chopped parsley

- 1 tablespoon olive oil

- 2 tablespoons lemon juice

- Salt and pepper to taste

Preparation Instructions:

1. In a medium bowl, combine the cooked lentils and quinoa.

2. Add in the chopped red onion, red bell pepper, and parsley.

3. Drizzle the olive oil and lemon juice over the salad and mix them together.

4. Add salt and pepper to the food to taste.

5. Serve chilled or at room temperature. Enjoy!

SNACK: Celery sticks with tahini

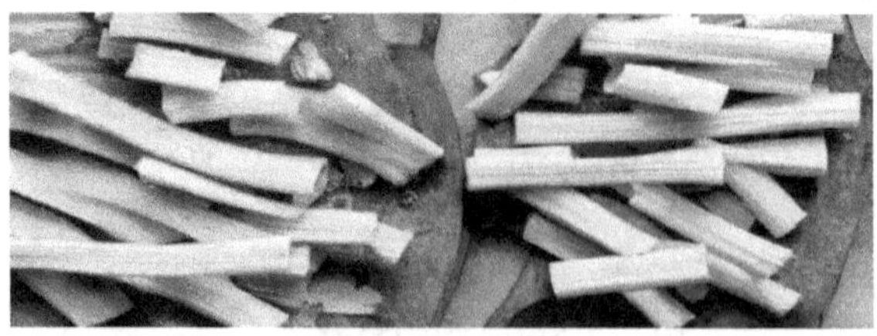

Prep Time: 10 minutes

GI Range: Low

Calorie Count: 100 calories per serving

Ingredients:

-2 stalks of celery, washed and cut into sticks

-1 tablespoon of tahini

-1 teaspoon of lemon juice

-1/4 teaspoon of garlic powder

-Salt and pepper to taste

Preparation Instructions:

1. In a small bowl, mix together the tahini, lemon juice, garlic powder, salt, and pepper.

2. Dip each celery stick into the tahini mixture, making sure to coat all sides.

3. Place the celery sticks on a plate and serve. Enjoy!

DINNER: Baked chicken with roasted vegetables

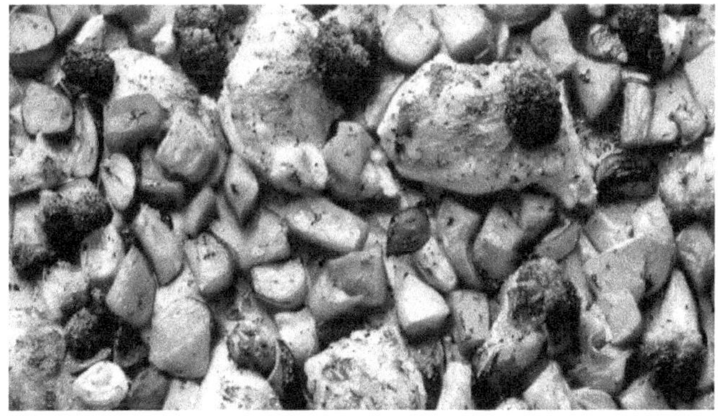

Prep Time: 30 minutes

GI Range: Low

Calorie Count: 400 Calories

Ingredients:

- 2 chicken breasts

- 2 tablespoons olive oil

- 1 teaspoon garlic powder

- 1 teaspoon onion powder

- 1 teaspoon dried oregano

- Salt and pepper to taste

- 2 cups mixed vegetables (e.g., broccoli, bell peppers, mushrooms, zucchini, carrots, etc.)

- 2 tablespoons balsamic vinegar

- 2 tablespoons fresh chopped herbs (e.g., oregano, thyme, parsley, etc.)

Preparation Instructions:

1. Preheat the oven to 400°F.

2. Place the chicken breasts on a baking sheet and season with garlic powder, onion powder, oregano, salt, and pepper. 1 tablespoon of olive oil should be drizzled on.

3. Bake the chicken for 15-20 minutes, or until cooked

through.

4. Meanwhile, in a large bowl, combine the vegetables with the remaining tablespoon of olive oil, balsamic vinegar, and herbs. Spread vegetables onto a separate baking sheet.

5. Place the vegetables in the oven and bake for 15-20 minutes, or until tender.

6. Serve chicken and vegetables together. Enjoy!

DAY 7

BREAKFAST: Banana, almond milk, and spinach smoothie

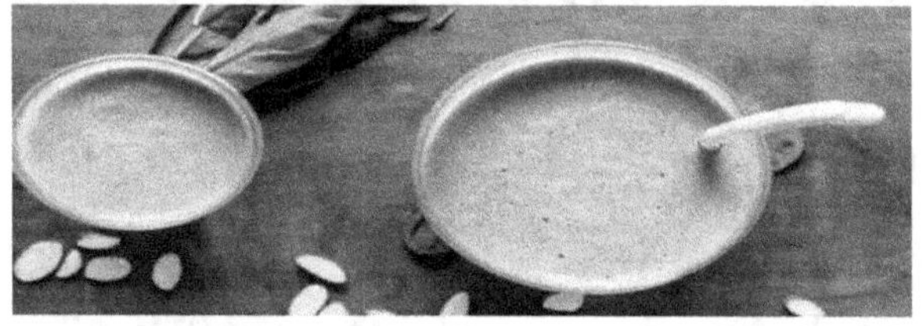

Prep Time: 10 minutes

GI range: Low

Calorie Count: 220

Ingredients:

- 2 ripe bananas
- 1 cup almond milk
- 1 cup spinach
- 2 tablespoons raw honey
- 1 teaspoon vanilla extract
- 1/2 cup ice

Preparation Instructions:

1. Peel and slice the bananas.

2. Place all ingredients in a blender.

3. Blend on high until smooth.

4. Serve cold.

SNACK: Air-popped popcorn

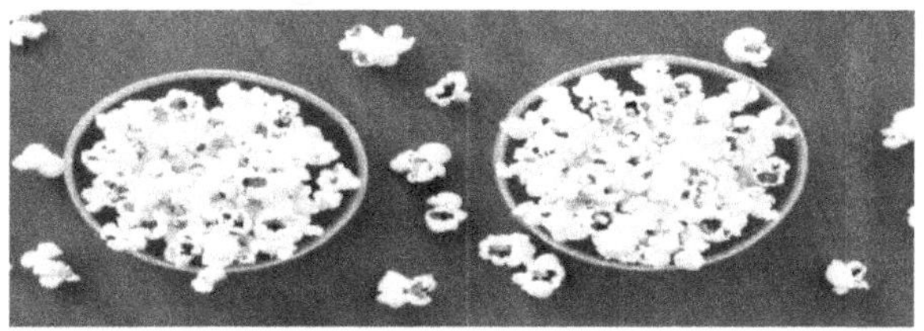

Prep Time: 5 minutes

GI Range: Low

Calorie Count: Approximately 30 calories per cup

Ingredients:

- 1/2 cup popcorn kernels
- 1 tablespoon cooking oil (avocado, olive, or coconut oil work best)
- Salt and pepper to taste

Preparation Instructions:

1. Heat a medium to a large pot over medium-high heat.

2. Add the cooking oil and allow it to heat up for a minute.

3. Add the popcorn kernels and stir to coat them in the oil.

4. Cover the pot and wait for the popcorn to start popping.

5. Once the popping has slowed down to a few kernels

per second, remove the pot from the heat and transfer the popcorn to a large bowl.

6. Sprinkle salt and pepper to taste, and enjoy!

LUNCH: Kale and white bean soup

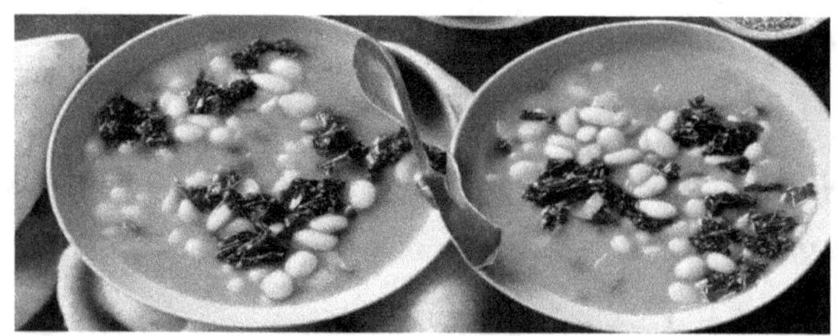

Prep Time: 45 minutes

GI Range: Low GI

Calorie Count: 160 calories per serving

Ingredients:

-1 tablespoon olive oil

-1 small onion, diced

-3 cloves garlic, minced

-4 cups vegetable broth

-1 (15.5 ounces) can of cannellini beans, drained and rinsed

-1 (14.5 ounces) can of diced tomatoes

-1/4 teaspoon dried oregano

-1/4 teaspoon dried thyme

-1/4 teaspoon dried basil

-1/4 teaspoon freshly ground black pepper

-2 cups chopped fresh kale

-1/4 cup freshly grated Parmesan cheese

Preparation Instructions:

1. Over medium heat, warm the olive oil in a big saucepan. Add onion and garlic and sauté until soft and fragrant, about 5 minutes.

2. Pour in vegetable broth, beans, tomatoes, oregano, thyme, basil, and black pepper. Boil for a little while, then turn down the heat and simmer for 30 minutes.

3. Add the kale and simmer for 10 more minutes.

4. Serve in bowls, topped with Parmesan cheese. Enjoy!

SNACK: Cucumber slices with cottage cheese

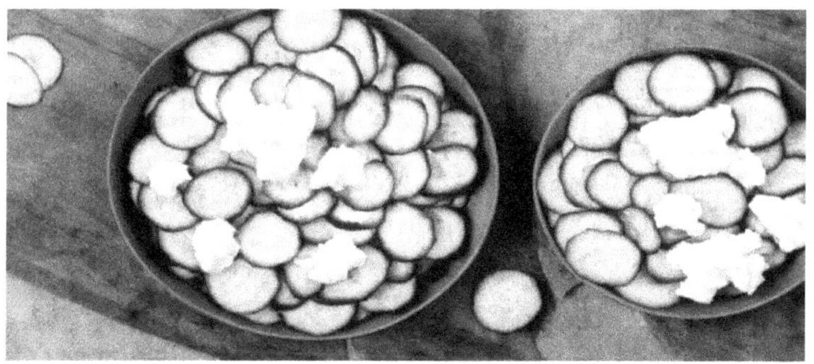

Prep Time: 10 minutes

Glycemic Index Range: Low

Calorie Count: Approximately 140 calories per serving

Ingredients:

- 1 cup of cottage cheese
- 2 large cucumbers, sliced
- Salt and pepper to taste
- 1 tablespoon of olive oil
- 1 tablespoon of lemon juice
- 1 tablespoon of chopped fresh parsley

Preparation Instructions:

1. Slice the cucumbers into 1/4-inch thick slices.

2. Place the cucumbers on a plate and season with salt and pepper.

3. In a small bowl, mix together the cottage cheese, olive oil, and lemon juice.

4. Spread the cottage cheese mixture onto the cucumber slices.

5. Sprinkle the chopped parsley onto the cucumber slices.

6. Serve immediately.

DINNER: Grilled steak with roasted sweet potatoes

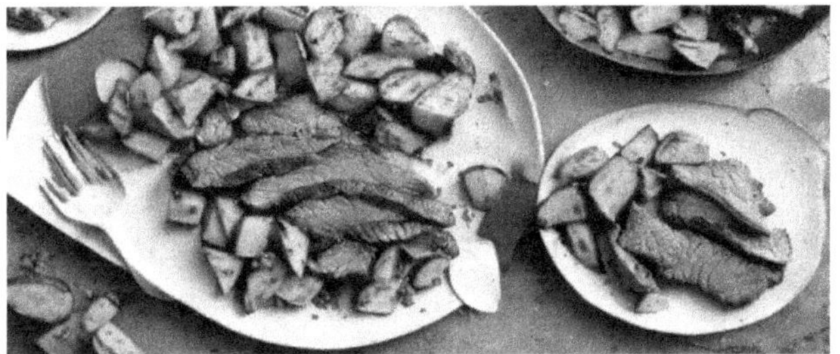

Prep Time: 30 minutes

GI Range: Very Low

Calorie Count: 350 calories

Ingredients:

-2 sirloin steaks

-2 sweet potatoes

-2 tablespoons olive oil

-1 teaspoon garlic powder

-1 teaspoon onion powder

-1 teaspoon cumin

-1 teaspoon smoked paprika

-Salt and pepper to taste

Preparation Instructions:

1. Preheat your grill to medium-high heat.

2. Peel and cube the sweet potatoes and place them in a bowl. Add the olive oil, garlic powder, onion powder,

cumin, smoked paprika, salt, and pepper. Toss to combine.

3. Place the seasoned sweet potatoes on the preheated grill and cook for 15 minutes, flipping once, until tender.

4. While the sweet potatoes are cooking, season the steaks with salt and pepper.

5. Grill the steaks for 4-5 minutes per side, or until desired doneness.

6. Serve the steak and roasted sweet potatoes together. Enjoy!

CONCLUSION

The glycemic index diet is a great option for those looking to maintain a healthy lifestyle and achieve a balanced diet. It is easy to understand and follow, and it won't require any drastic changes to your current eating habits. By controlling your carbohydrate intake and focusing on low-GI foods, you can easily control your blood sugar levels and enjoy a wide variety of delicious, healthy meals. This diet also emphasizes the importance of portion control and regular exercise, which can help you reach and maintain your desired weight. Overall, the glycemic index diet is an excellent choice for anyone looking to improve their health and wellbeing. With its simple guidelines and focus on nutritious, low-GI foods, it can help you reach your goals and enjoy a healthier lifestyle.

Happy Cooking!

BONUS:

30-DAY

MEAL PLANNER

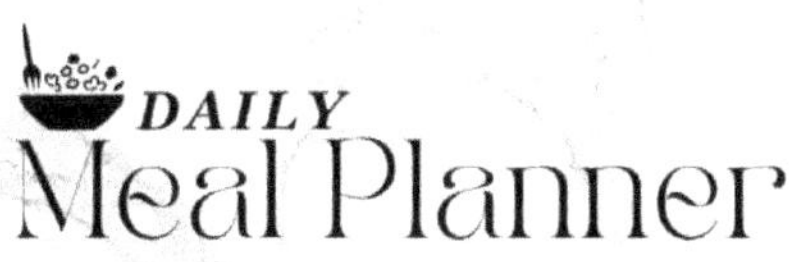

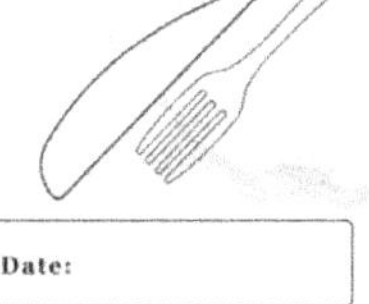

Date:

Breakfast

Grocery List

Lunch

Dinner

Snack

NOTES:

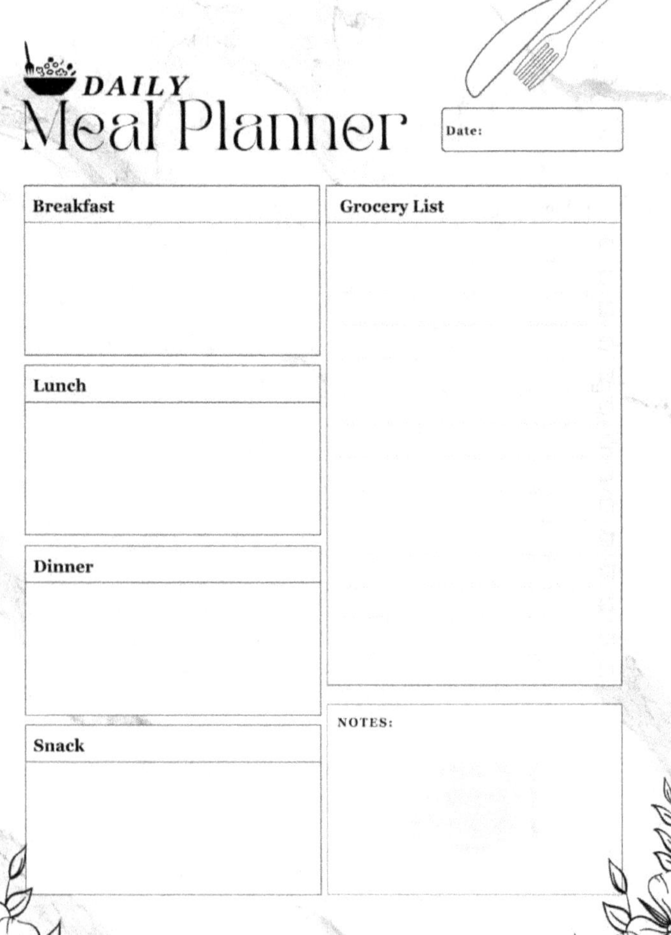
DAILY
Meal Planner
Date:
Breakfast
Lunch
Dinner
Snack
Grocery List
NOTES:

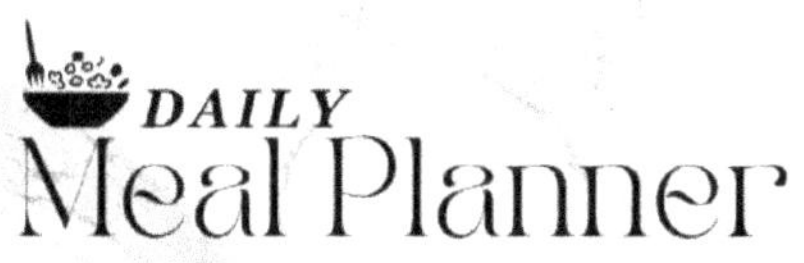

DAILY
Meal Planner

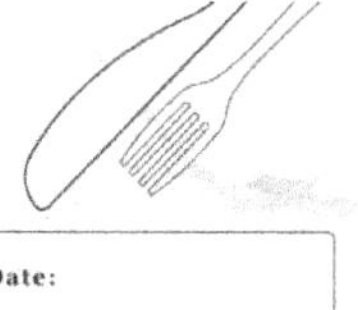

Date:

Breakfast

Lunch

Dinner

Snack

Grocery List

NOTES:

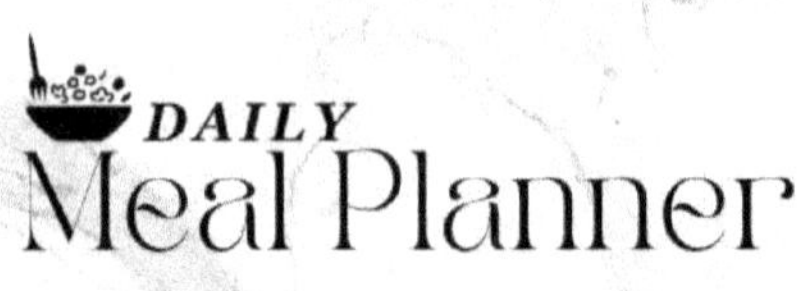

DAILY
Meal Planner

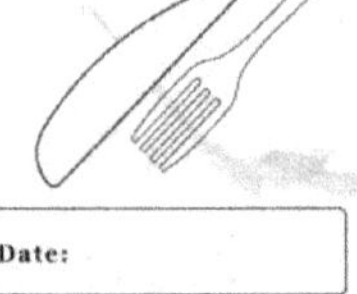

Date:

Breakfast

Lunch

Dinner

Snack

Grocery List

NOTES:

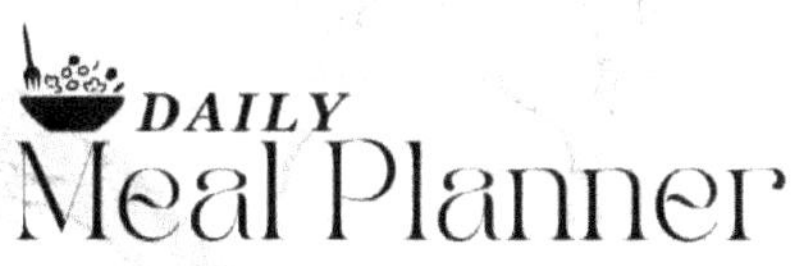

DAILY Meal Planner

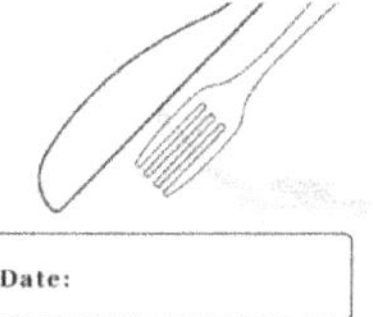

Date:

Breakfast

Lunch

Dinner

Snack

Grocery List

NOTES:

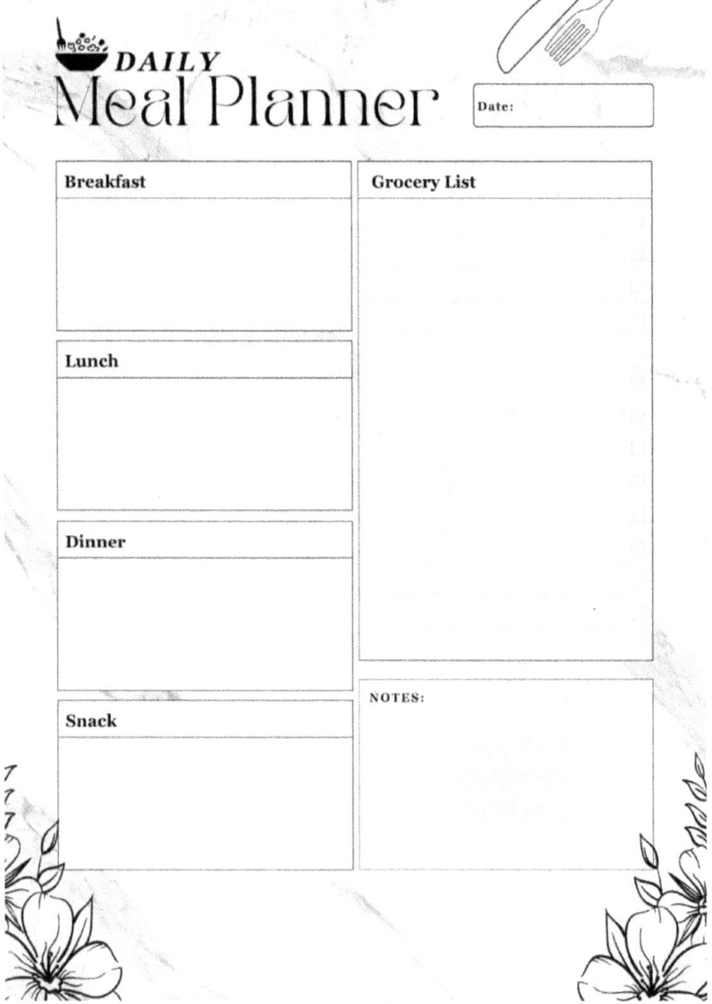

DAILY
Meal Planner
Date:
Breakfast
Grocery List
Lunch
Dinner
Snack
NOTES:

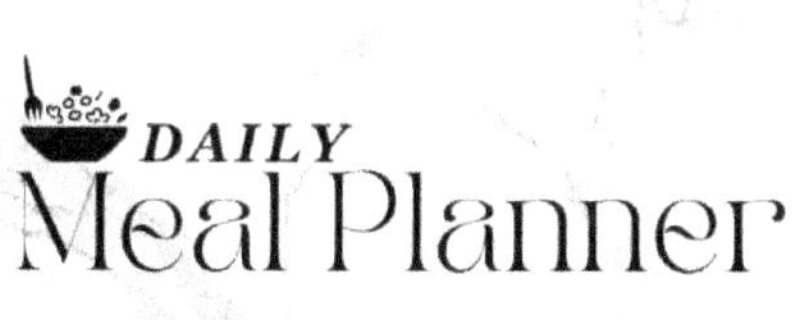
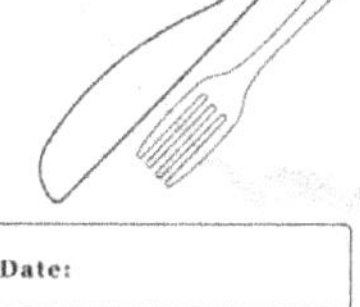

DAILY
Meal Planner

Date:

Breakfast

Lunch

Dinner

Snack

Grocery List

NOTES:

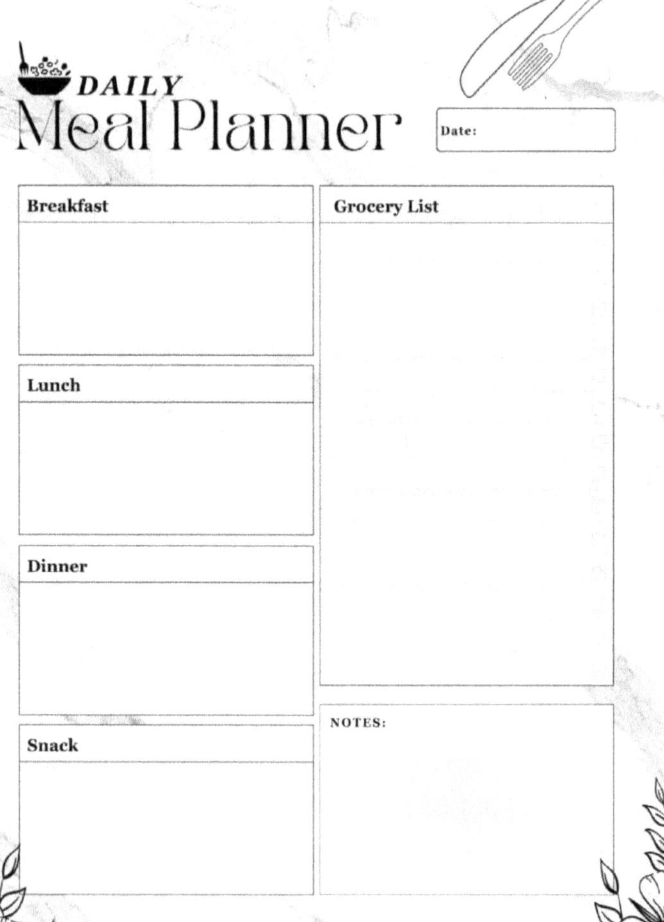
DAILY
Meal Planner
Date:
Breakfast
Lunch
Dinner
Snack
Grocery List
NOTES:

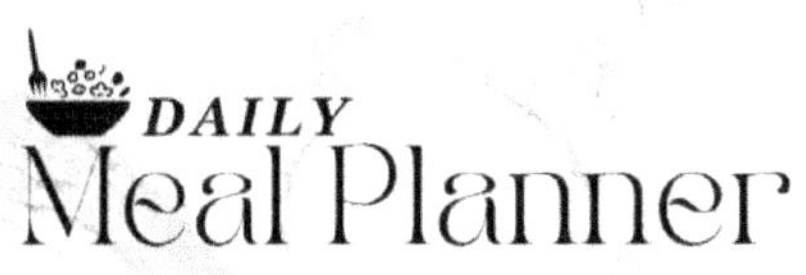
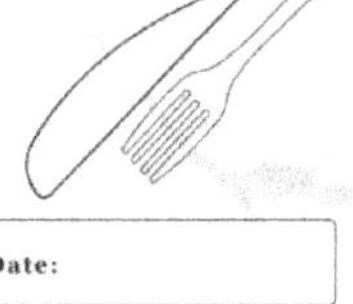

DAILY
Meal Planner

Date:

Breakfast

Lunch

Dinner

Snack

Grocery List

NOTES:

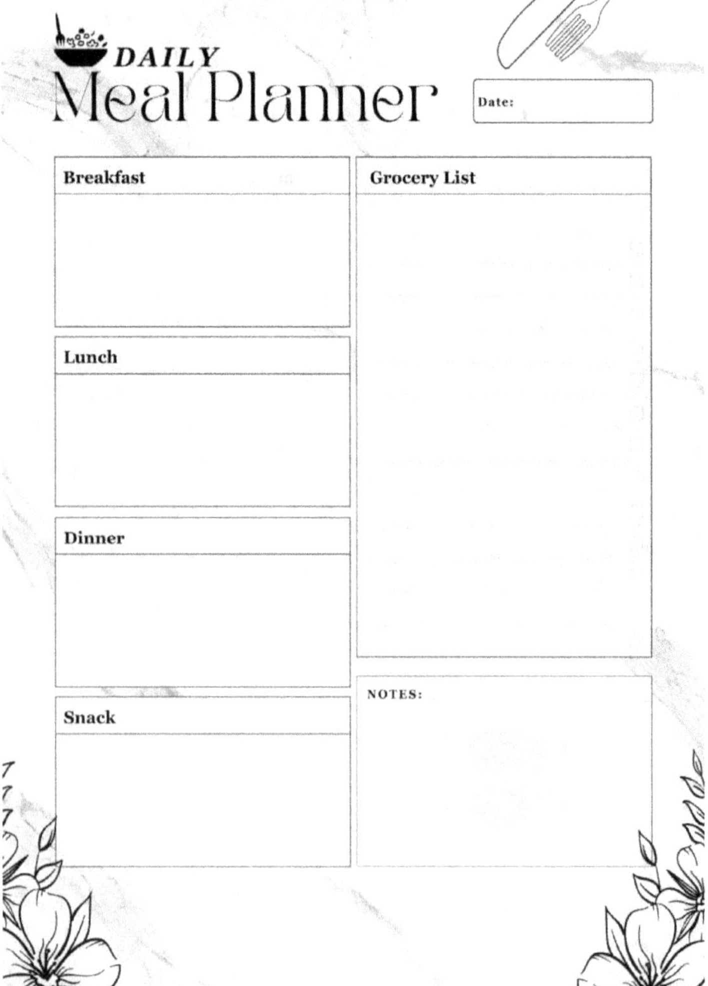
DAILY
Meal Planner
Date:
Breakfast
Grocery List
Lunch
Dinner
Snack
NOTES:

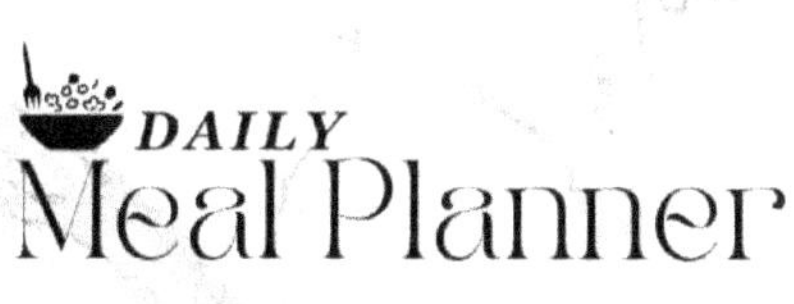 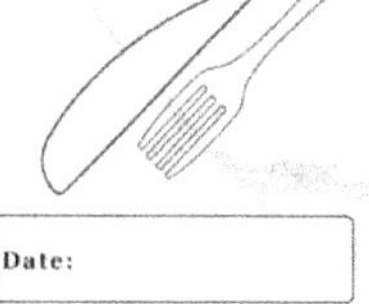

DAILY
Meal Planner

Date:

Breakfast

Lunch

Dinner

Snack

Grocery List

NOTES:

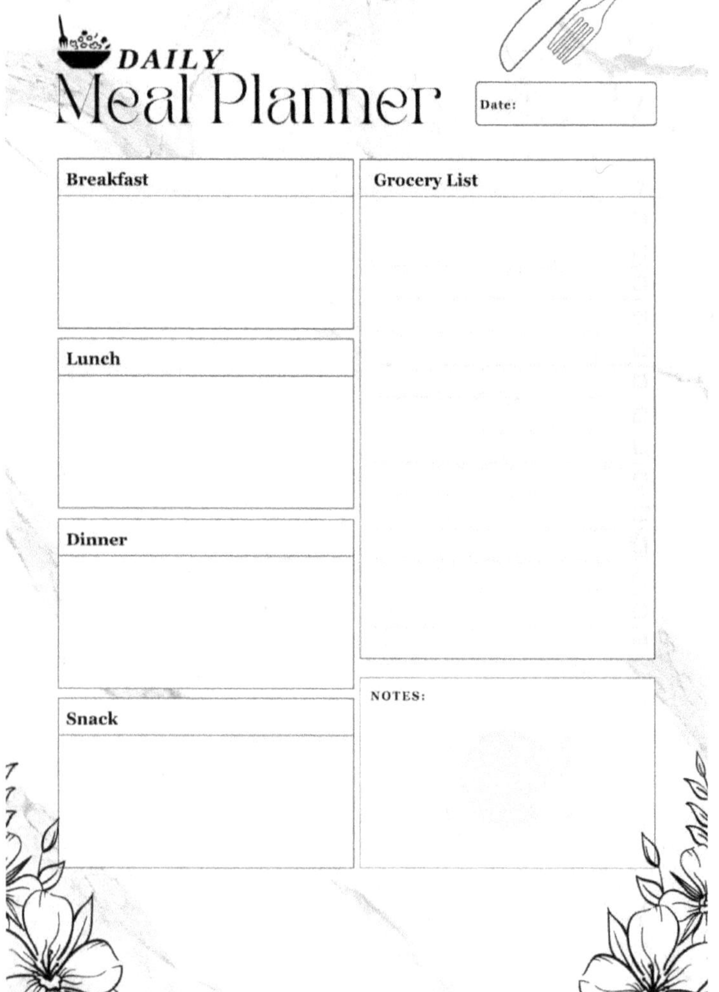
DAILY
Meal Planner
Date:
Breakfast
Lunch
Dinner
Snack
Grocery List
NOTES:

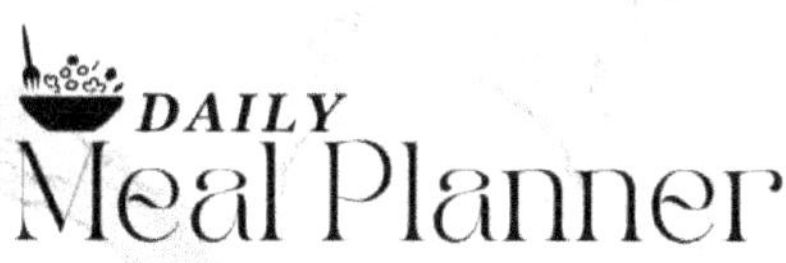
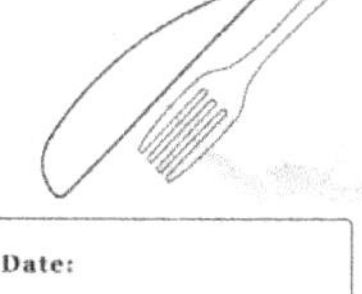

DAILY Meal Planner

Date:

Breakfast

Lunch

Dinner

Snack

Grocery List

NOTES:

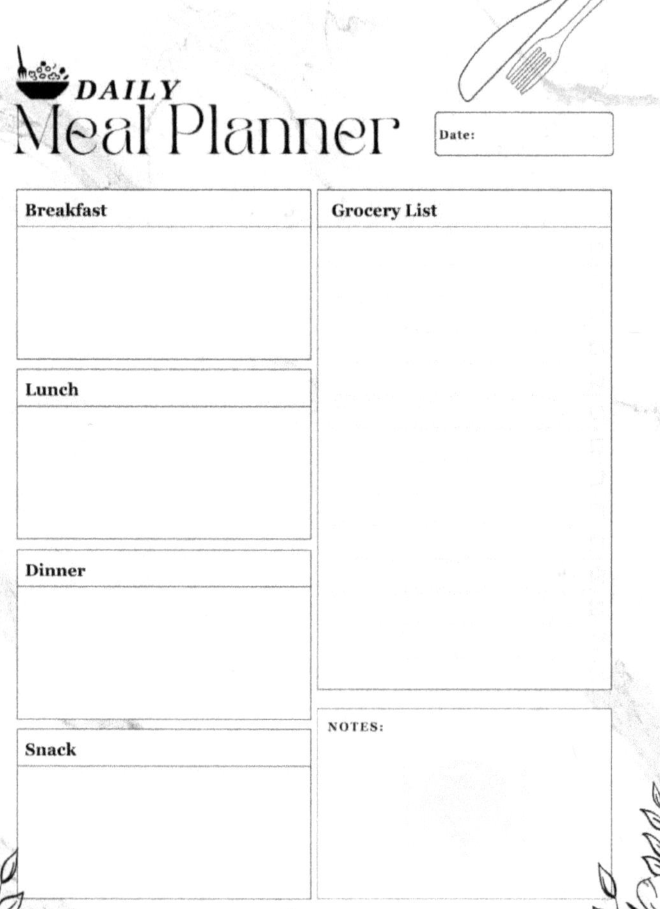
DAILY
Meal Planner
Date:
Breakfast
Lunch
Dinner
Snack
Grocery List
NOTES:

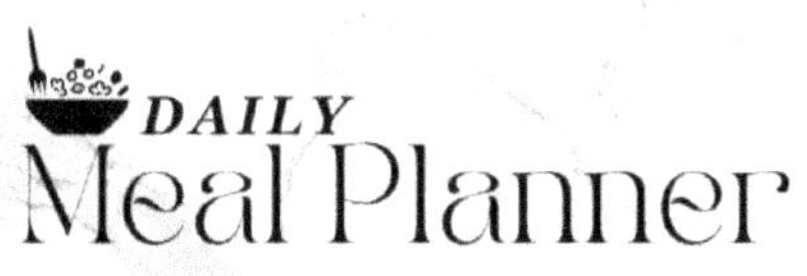

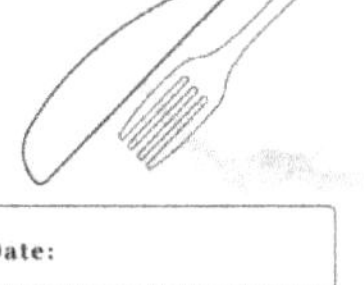

Date:

Breakfast

Grocery List

Lunch

Dinner

Snack

NOTES:

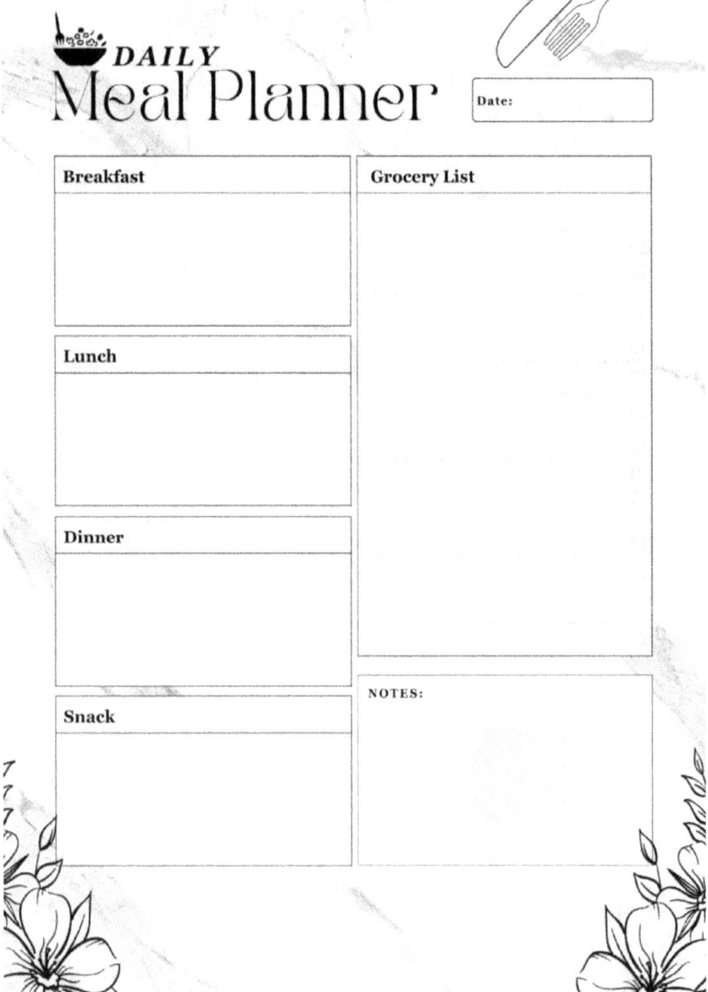

DAILY
Meal Planner
Date:
Breakfast
Lunch
Dinner
Snack
Grocery List
NOTES:

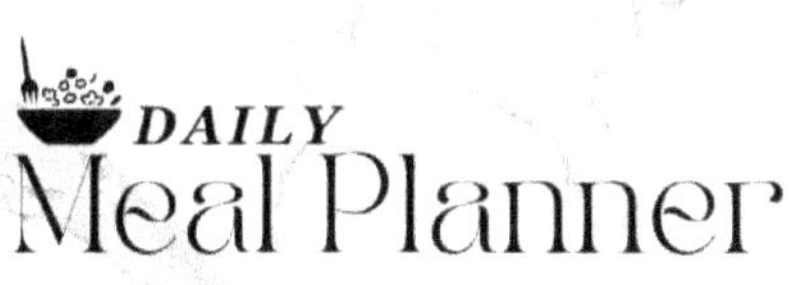

DAILY
Meal Planner

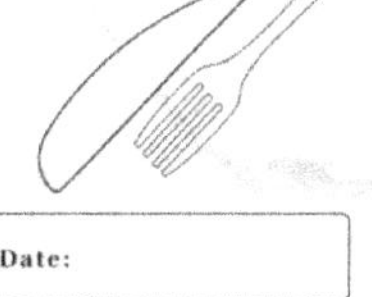

Date:

Breakfast

Grocery List

Lunch

Dinner

Snack

NOTES:

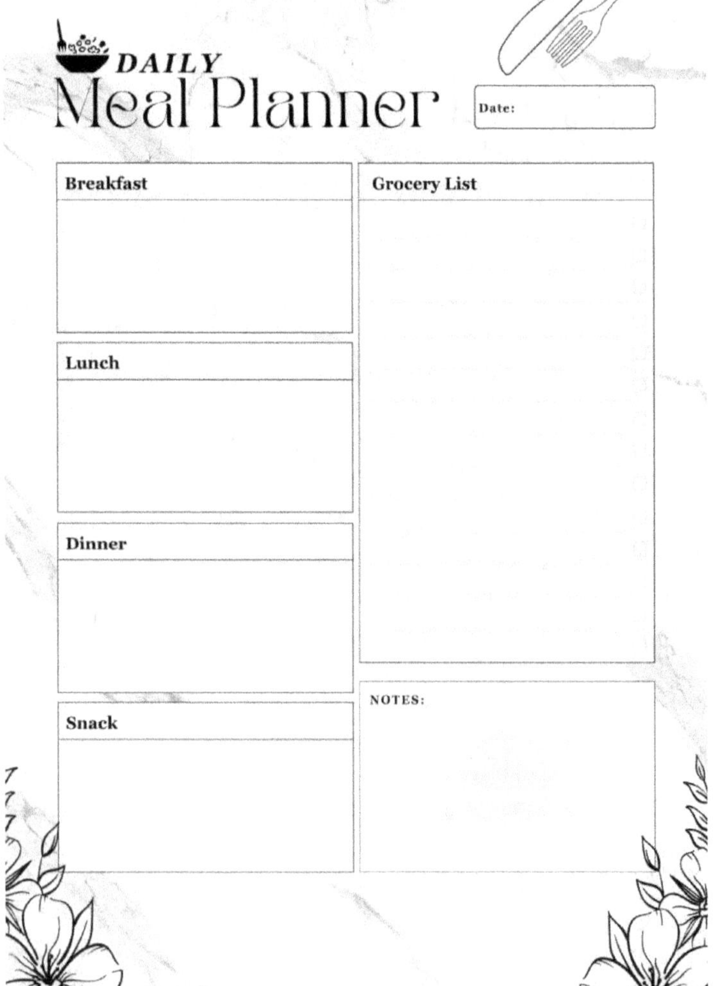

DAILY
Meal Planner
Date:
Breakfast
Lunch
Dinner
Snack
Grocery List
NOTES:

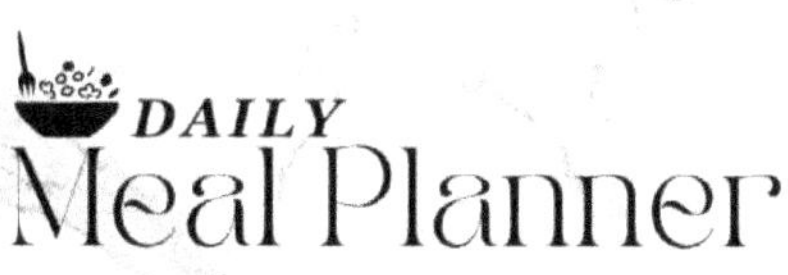 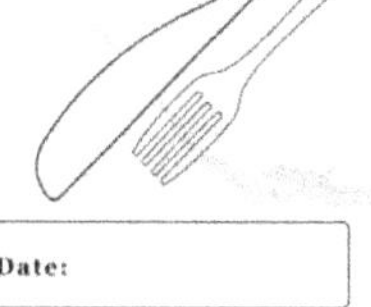

DAILY
Meal Planner

Date:

Breakfast

Lunch

Dinner

Snack

Grocery List

NOTES:

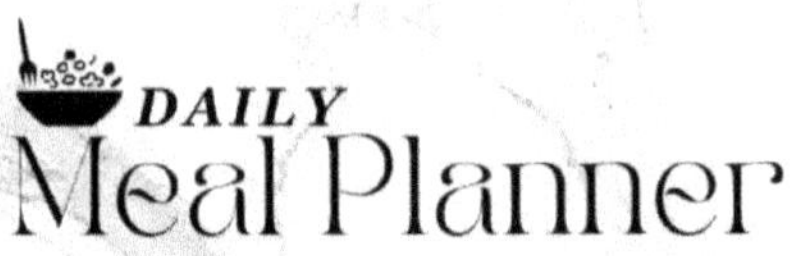 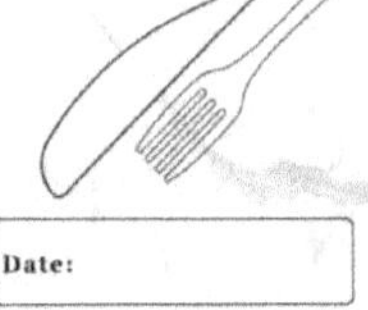

DAILY
Meal Planner

Date:

Breakfast

Lunch

Dinner

Snack

Grocery List

NOTES:

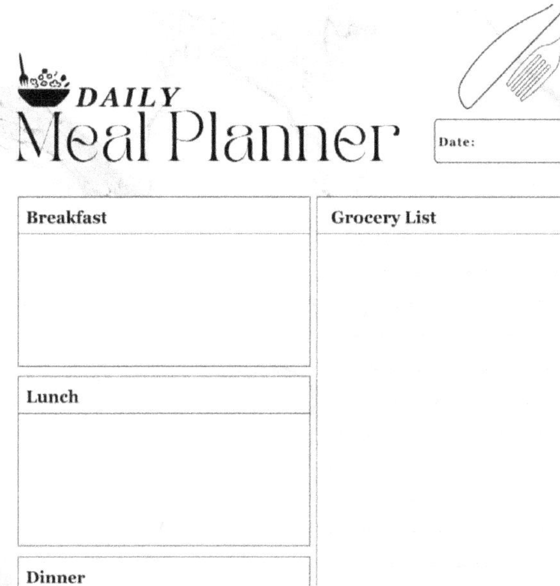
DAILY
Meal Planner
Date:
Breakfast
Lunch
Dinner
Snack
Grocery List
NOTES:

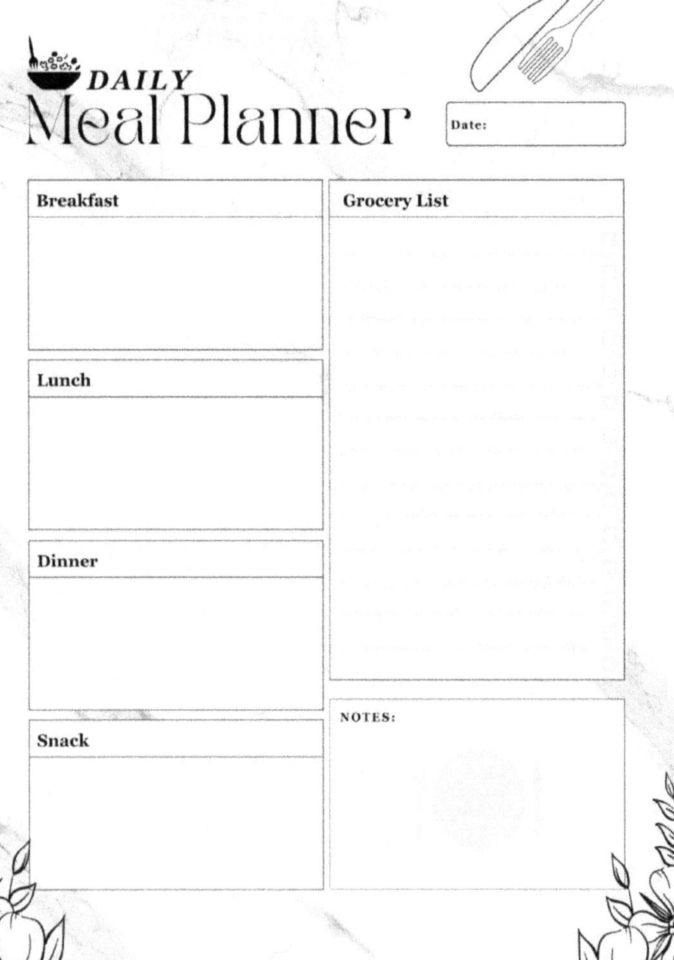
DAILY
Meal Planner
Date:
Breakfast
Lunch
Dinner
Snack
Grocery List
NOTES:

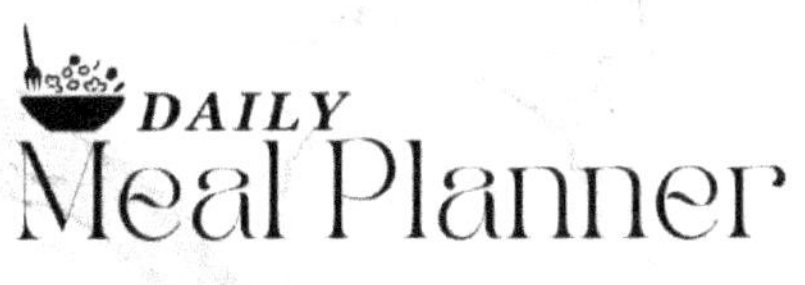

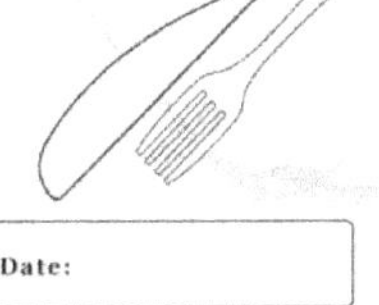

DAILY

Meal Planner

Date:

Breakfast

Grocery List

Lunch

Dinner

Snack

NOTES:

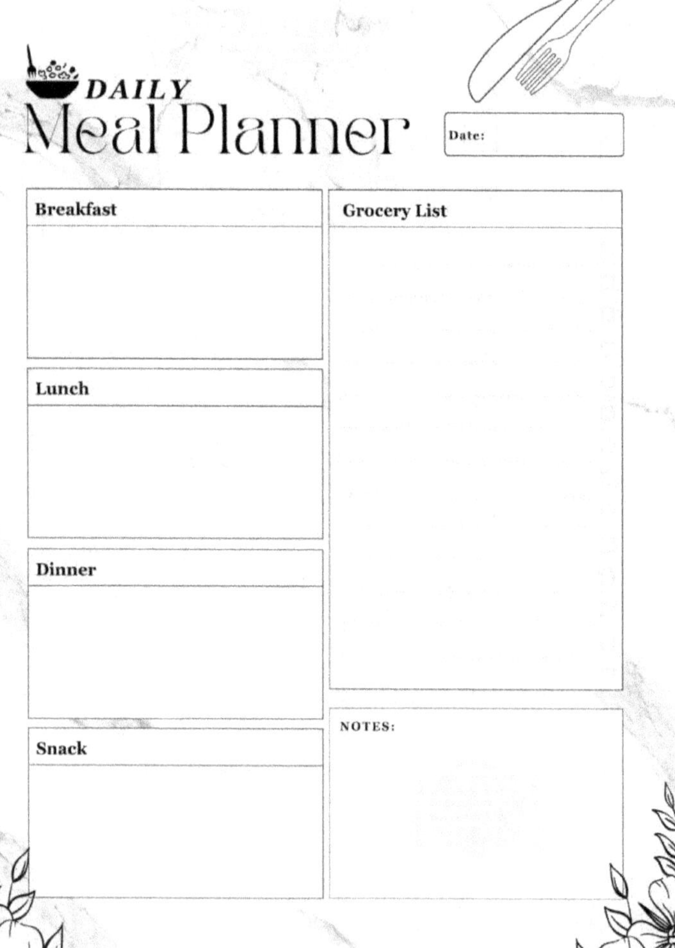
DAILY
Meal Planner
Date:
Breakfast
Lunch
Dinner
Snack
Grocery List
NOTES:

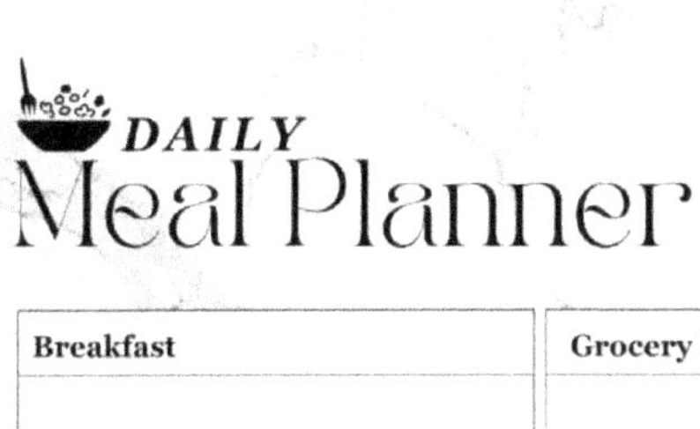

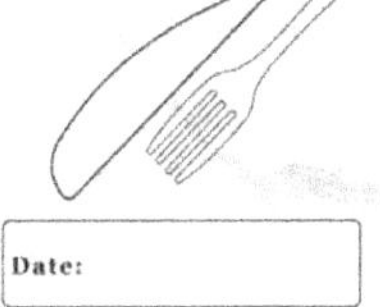

Date:

Breakfast

Lunch

Dinner

Snack

Grocery List

NOTES:

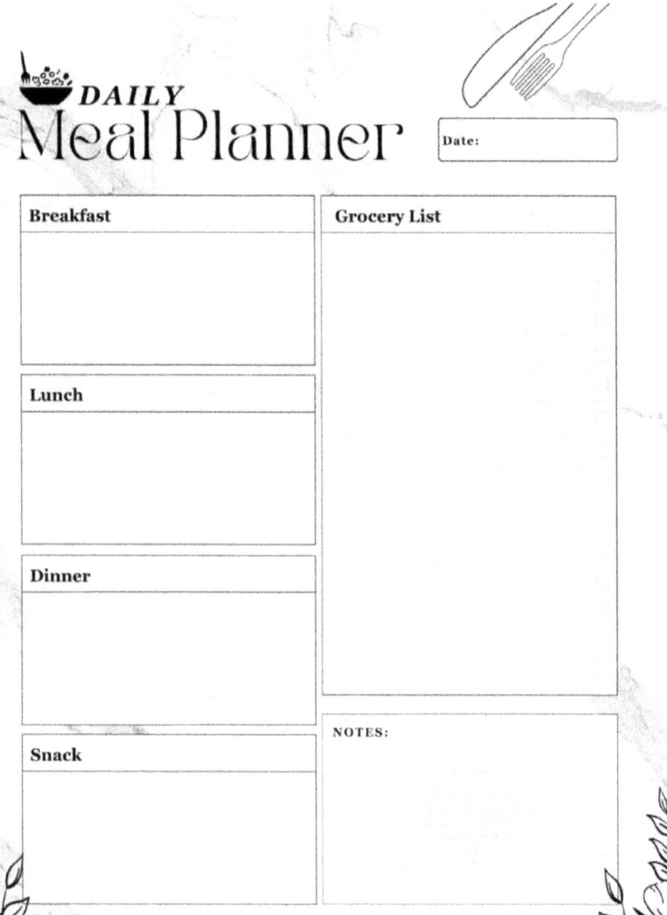
DAILY
Meal Planner
Date:
Breakfast
Lunch
Dinner
Snack
Grocery List
NOTES:

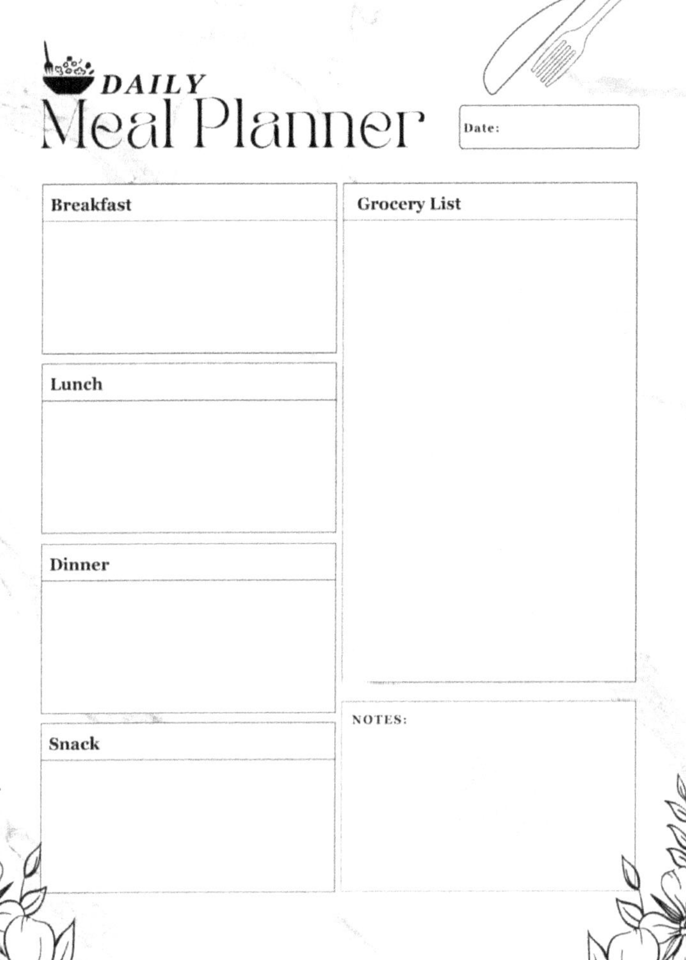
DAILY
Meal Planner
Date:
Breakfast
Lunch
Dinner
Snack
Grocery List
NOTES:

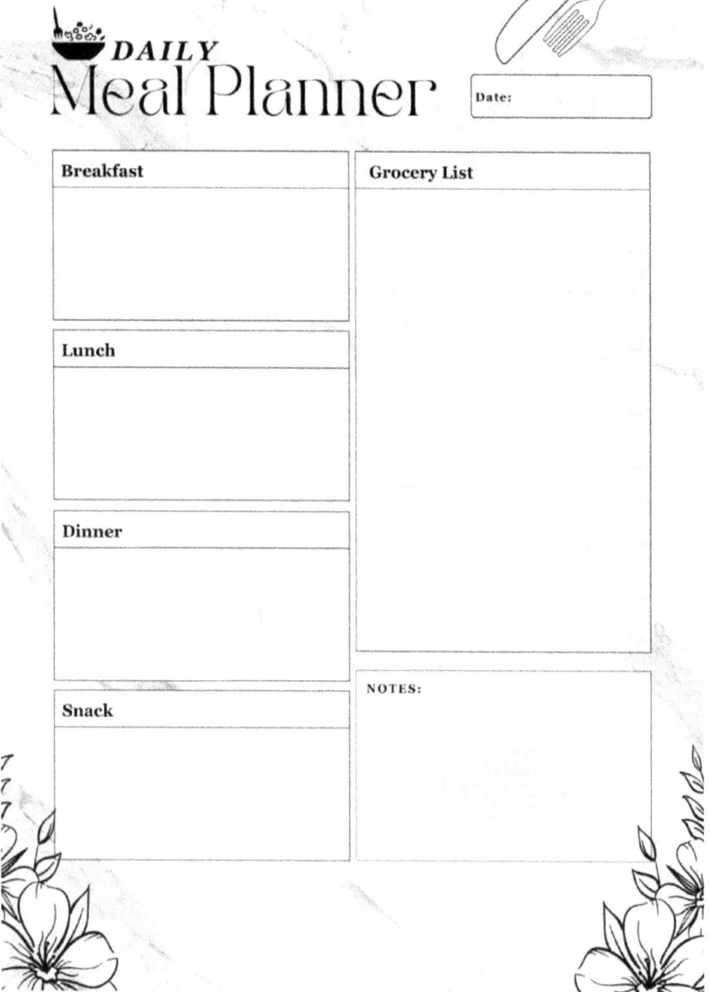

DAILY
Meal Planner
Date:
Breakfast
Lunch
Dinner
Snack
Grocery List
NOTES:

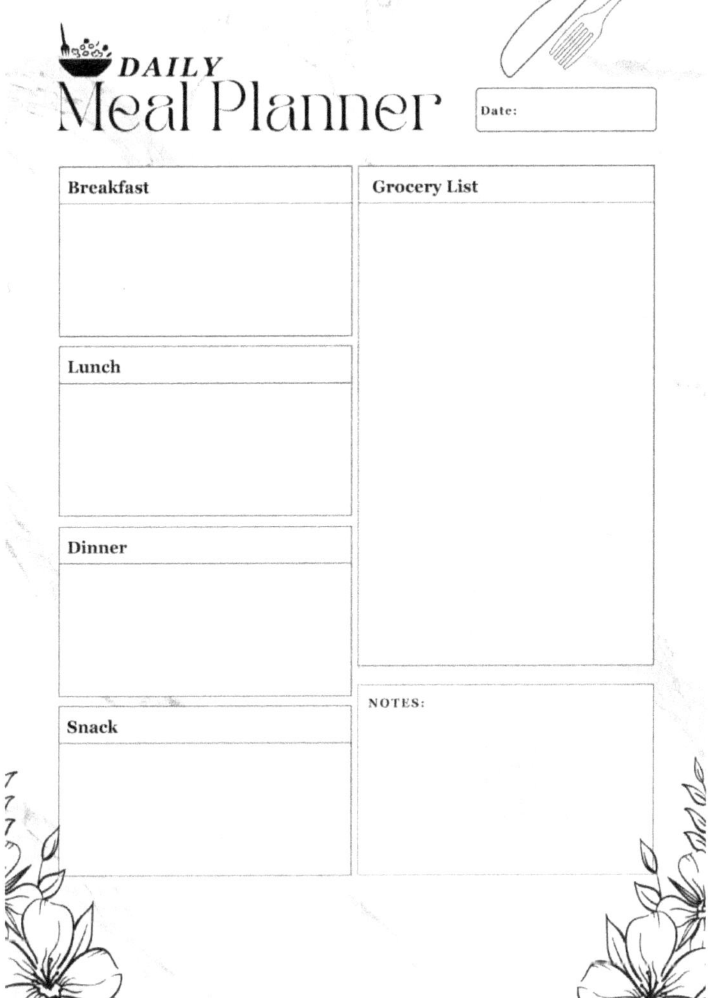
DAILY
Meal Planner
Date:
Breakfast
Lunch
Dinner
Snack
Grocery List
NOTES:

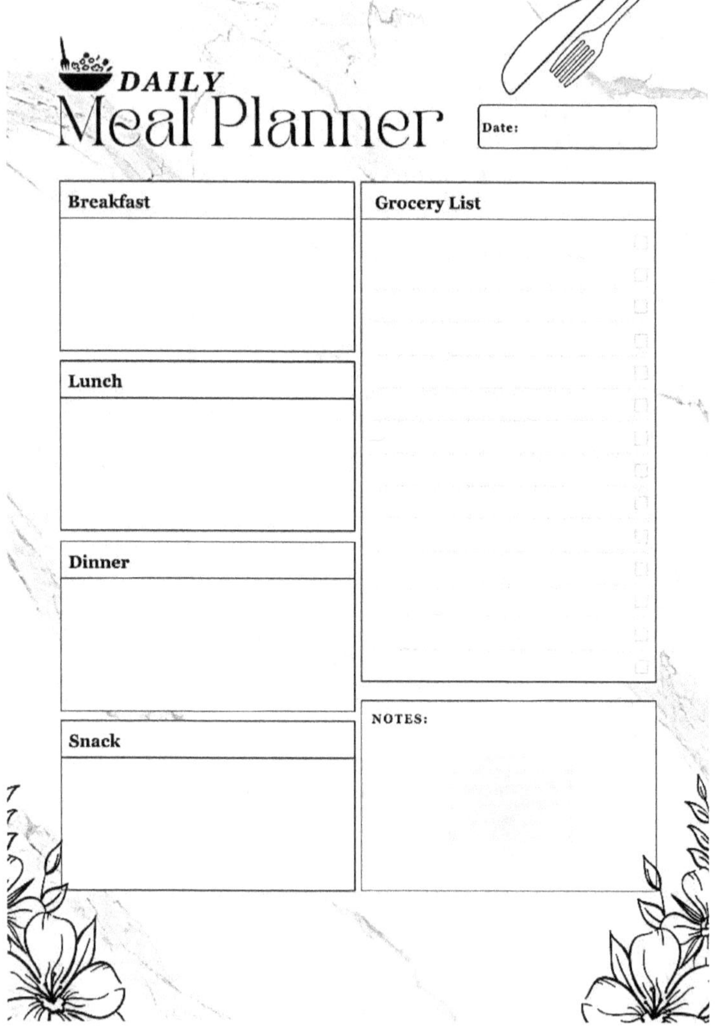

DAILY
Meal Planner
Date:
Breakfast
Lunch
Dinner
Snack
Grocery List
NOTES: